CONVERSATIONS WITH MY DAUGHTER

HOW TO HAVE A
HEALTHY
BABY

DAGMAR GANSER

Copyright © 2023 Dagmar Ganser. All rights reserved.

No part of this book may be used, transmitted, or reproduced in any form or by any means, graphic, electronic, or mechanical, including photocopying, recording, taping or by any information storage retrieval system without the written permission of the author except in the case of brief quotations embodied in critical articles and reviews. Because of the dynamic nature of the Internet, any web addresses or links contained in this book may have changed since publication and may no longer be valid.

DISCLAIMER:
The author of this book does not dispense medical advice or prescribe the use of any technique as a form of treatment for physical, emotional, or medical problems without the advice of a physician, either directly or indirectly. The intent of the author is only to offer information of a general nature to help you in your quest for emotional and spiritual well-being. In the event you use any of the information in this book for yourself, which is your constitutional right, the author assumes no responsibility for your actions. Every attempt has been made to provide accurate and effective information; the author and this book do not guarantee results.

With the best of intention, 'female' or 'woman' refers to people assigned female at birth (AFAB). Likewise 'male' or 'man' refers to people assigned male at birth (AMAB). Please know that although the correct language is challenging to represent at every opportunity, inclusivity and diversity is highly valued and at the heart of all the information provided.

Certain stock imagery © Getty Images.
Graphic Design: Anders Bundgaard
Edited by: Balboa.Press

ISBN: 978-0-6459067-0-7 (sc)
ISBN: 978-0-6459067-1-4 (e)
rev. date: 21 August 2023

True Medicine
PO Box 900, Sanctuary Cove Qld 4212, Australia
www.truemedicine.com.au

CONTENTS

About this Book vii
Foreword ix
Introduction xi
Reasons for Infertility xiii

Section I   Preparation xv

Chapter 1   Let's Begin with the Men 1
Chapter 2   Your Turn, Ladies 9
Chapter 3   Sperm Meets Egg 15
Chapter 4   Environmental Toxins 20
Chapter 5   Diet 42
Chapter 6   The B Vitamins 49
Chapter 7   Genes and Epigenetics 55
Chapter 8   Gut health 62
Chapter 9   The Importance of Water 67
Chapter 10   Final Steps of Preparation 70

Section II   Conception 73

Chapter 11   Ready for Conception 75
Chapter 12   Nutrition for Mother and Baby 77
Chapter 13   Pregnancy Woes 84
Chapter 14   Preparing for Birth 89

Section III   Birth 93

Chapter 15   Congratulations on Your New Baby 95
Chapter 16   Time for Solid Food 100
Chapter 17   Skin and Other Irritations 106
Chapter 18   Baby's Emotional Foundations 110
Chapter 19   The Baby Blues 112
Chapter 20   Stress 115
Chapter 21   Oxidative Stress 124

Chapter 22 Post Baby Recovery 126
Chapter 23 Preventative Medicine 128
Appendix 1 Diet Guidelines.. 131
Appendix 2 Nutrition Guidelines... 137
Appendix 3 Labs and Tests Guide.. 155
Appendix 4 Suppliers.. 159
Appendix 5 Recommended Reading 161

Glossary.. 163
Acknowledgements 173
Permissions.. 175
Sources and References 177

ABOUT THIS BOOK

There is nothing more precious than a new life. The excitement of conception turns into wonder as the tiny speck inside a woman's womb grows into a baby. Our wonder does not diminish as we watch that baby grow into a toddler, learning how to walk and navigate its way through life. Giving the gift of life is an honour, and it is our responsibility to ensure the child we create has every opportunity to lead a long and healthy life.

Making a baby sounds relatively simple—egg plus sperm and, about forty weeks later, a baby is born. For many couples this dream seems unachievable and can lead to feelings of inadequacy and bitter disappointment. In Australia between 15 and 18 per cent of couples are infertile, with about one in six couples experiencing fertility issues and up to 25 per cent of all pregnancies ending in miscarriage. Whether you are seeking to conceive naturally, with the help of assisted reproductive technologies (ART), in-vitro fertilisation (IVF), or with the help of a surrogate or donor, the information in this book will greatly assist in you achieving that dream. If you have been experiencing any fertility issues, this book will provide answers and tools to help you achieve your dream of having a baby.

But *How to have a Healthy Baby* deals with more than fertility—it's about having a *healthy* baby. It's about helping you understand the impacts of our modern way of life, including environmental toxins, stress, lifestyle, and low-nutrient diets, on fertility and conception. This book will give you power through understanding the role you play in, not only conceiving but also nourishing your baby while in utero, birthing a healthy child, and ensuring that child grows into a healthy adult. The book is divided into three sections—preparation, conception and pregnancy, and birth. Each section explains easy steps you can take to support your health, optimise fertility, and have a *healthy* baby.

Conversations with My Daughter: How to have a Healthy Baby is an illuminating journey into the workings of the human body and how we all have the power to give ourselves and our children the best chance at health and vitality.

FOREWORD

Raising healthy children is the most important job in the world. No other act has a more permanent, lasting impact on the world around us than does the raising of children. In the natural sciences, we judge the health of animal populations by the productivity and success of the parents in raising healthy offspring. It is easy to understand, and simple to observe, that a species that struggles to successfully breed and produce offspring is a species under threat. This is something grade school children the world over learn about our natural world. And yet it's an idea we take for granted and one that too often goes unexamined. For some reason, we tend to think that producing healthy offspring in animals is somehow different than the conceiving, birthing, and raising of children. But is it really that different?

As humans, we sit atop creation with an unmatched set of problem-solving tools, language, art, and cognitive ability. Yet, on the biological and cellular level, we are still very much an animal. So, when we look at the challenges facing our species—the human family—in the same way we look at a species of frog or bird of prey, we can see some very concerning warning signs. We are experiencing rapid increases in the rates of infertility in women, while the levels of testosterone and sperm, markers of biological male fitness, are in a state of rapid decline. Children are struggling with chronic diseases and challenging diagnoses that were unheard of just a generation prior. Kids are experiencing stroke, cardiovascular disease, obesity, diabetes, sensory processing disorders, and allergies at levels beyond anything we have ever seen before.

The answer to this epidemic of sick children and frustrated and broken-hearted parents is to get healthy before you get pregnant. The way to do that in today's stressful, toxic world is to optimise the terrain inside your own body. You don't have to get a PhD in nutrition, genetics, or biochemistry, but you do have to relearn some things and unlearn some others. The methylation pathway, and the MTHFR gene, is probably the most important pathway for moms-to-be (and dads-to-be) to optimise before they start a family. Luckily, you will learn about this and many other related ideas in the pages to come.

This book is an important guide for moms and dads to make the important, long-lasting changes necessary to promote an optimum pregnancy. We all want to have healthy children, but that healthy child first starts with a healthy pregnancy. This epidemic of infertility and childhood illness share a common cause of stress, toxicity, and malnutrition. And if this common cause is addressed by responsible parents-to-be before starting a family, massive positive changes can be made to alleviate the risks of these frustrating health problems.

Lastly, if it was easy, everyone would do it! How many people do you know who began to detoxify their bodies and improve their nutrition, reduce their stress, optimise their sleep and exercise, and do a dozen other healthy habits every day … six months before they even started trying to have a family? Probably not very many. We need parents to put the work in early, before conception, throughout the pregnancy and into the early years. If you follow the information in this book, we can create a world full of healthy children, moms, and dads. And that is a world worth working towards.

Dr Andrew Rostenberg, DC, DIBAK

INTRODUCTION

This book has been many years in the making. When my eldest daughter moved back home in her late twenties, we were able to spend more time together. All too often while chatting over breakfast, she asked why I didn't write a book to share my knowledge. I had never considered myself an author, so I dismissed this suggestion. However, as the years passed and I witnessed with great sadness the ever-growing incidence of poor health—particularly in children—the seed began to sprout.

It is heart-wrenching to witness a baby, toddler, or child suffering due to ill health. During the past twenty years in clinic, I have witnessed far too many young children suffering with pain or inability to do things their friends can do.

So, here I go with the book suggested by my beautiful daughter—empowering you with knowledge that will help you understand all the complexities we face in our modern lives and how these affect the health of our children. The only way to break the sickness continuum is right at the beginning—ensuring our babies are born healthy. The foundations for a healthy life are laid well before conception, and as every parent wants the best for their child, this book will both educate and inspire you to take a few easy steps towards this goal. By making a few simple shifts in your lifestyle and diet, you can positively influence the health of your child/children. Far too many children are growing up to experience avoidable illnesses—obesity, diabetes, behavioural issues, allergies, and heart disease, just to name a few.

The book will focus on and discuss the different stages in the process of having a baby. Section 1 outlines and explains modern-day challenges, which include environmental toxins and nutritional deficiencies. You will learn how genes and epigenetics play a role, followed by simple things you can do to ensure the best outcome for you and your baby. Conception is a truly amazing phenomenon, which you will appreciate even more in the chapter explaining what actually happens once fertilisation occurs. This will help you understand the utmost importance of preparation and ensuring that both parents are as healthy as they can possibly be.

After learning more about the role of natural medicine, diet, and lifestyle in ensuring that your baby gets the best start to life, you'll be ready to make your healthy baby. Section 2 focuses on gestation and how your needs, along with your baby's needs, change throughout the forty weeks. Once again, natural medicine offers some easy solutions to common concerns such as morning sickness and baby brain. Then we'll enter the first few months with your new baby and the challenges this period presents to all in the family, as well as evidence-based advice regarding your and your baby's nutrition.

I hope you have fun along the way while learning about this very serious topic. Every child is precious and deserves the very best start in life. After twenty years in clinical practice, it is high time I share some easy-to-follow tools to give you peace of mind and confidence that your child will have the best opportunity for a long and healthy life. So, let's begin the conversation and start working towards having a healthy baby.

REASONS FOR INFERTILITY

> Unexplained infertility generally means the physician failed
> to find the true cause of your infertility
> —Dr Norbert Gleicher

There are many contributing factors to infertility—both in men and women. While some of these factors apply to both genders, there are a few significant differences.

Women are born with all their oocytes (immature eggs or ova), whereas men produce sperm continuously from puberty onwards. While the oocytes are cocooned within the ovaries, they are still exposed to a myriad of environmental impacts, particularly while the female foetus is developing in her mother's womb. According to the 2015 Australian Institute of Health and Welfare report, babies are now more likely to be born to older mums.[1] As the age of conception rises, the duration of exposure to environmental toxins is prolonged.

This is one of the reasons many women experience problems conceiving once past the age of thirty-five but more so after the age of forty. But it's not all about women. Dr Michelle Wellman, a fertility specialist and surgical gynaecologist at Fertility SA, says that male fertility deteriorates later, after age thirty-five too, with older men less likely to conceive and some studies showing that the quality of sperm after forty years of age can contribute to genetic mutations.[1]

A recently released thirty-eight-year study showed that sperm count has declined significantly since the 1970s, which suggests both environmental and lifestyle factors. With increasing age, the risk of having a child with disabilities also increases.

So, what are some of the factors that affect fertility?

In both men and women, the common underlying factors include obesity, stress, environmental toxins, nutritional deficiencies, alcohol and caffeine consumption, systemic inflammation, low body fat, excessive exercise, smoking, imbalanced microbiome, glyphosate exposure, infection, insulin resistance, thyroid dysregulation, compromised detoxification, use of recreational/illicit or prescription drugs, radiation exposure and, specifically in women, endometriosis or polycystic ovarian syndrome (PCOS). These factors also contribute to adverse pregnancy outcomes and can increase the child's risk of disease later in life.

It is for this reason that the above issues must be addressed well before you want to start trying to fall pregnant. Actually, if you think you may want to start a family several years down the track, it is never too early to begin incorporating the suggestions contained in this book. According to a comprehensive survey of adult diets, the Australian Health Survey (ABS 2014) found that men and women of all ages were not meeting the recommended daily intake of each of the food groups.[2] The major food groups are protein, carbohydrates, and fats, as well as vitamins and minerals. Lifestyle and diet play a major role in your health and how your body functions, and therefore, both are especially relevant when seeking to have a healthy baby. I'll go into diet and nutrition later, but let's look at how you can best prepare your body.

It is not only the woman who needs to be aware of potential impediments to having a healthy baby. Men also need to prepare their body prior to conception to ensure their sperm fertilises the egg and produces a healthy baby. After all, the sperm delivers half of the genetic material required to make a baby. But sperm do so much more —the processes that occur during fertilisation are complex and rely on the sperm having all the "ingredients" required to start cell division. Sperm also play an essential role in the formation of the placenta and avoiding miscarriage.

> Failing to prepare is preparing to fail.
> —John Wooden

SECTION I
Preparation

Intellectuals solve problems,
geniuses prevent them.
—Unknown

1

Let's Begin with the Men

I am beginning with the man's role in making a baby because, when it comes to all things fertility, conception, and pregnancy, we mostly relate to women. However, the man plays a vital role in the process of having a healthy baby—and not just in a physical sense. Not only does the man contribute half of the genes that will make up the child's genome but his sperm influence fertilisation of the egg and formation of the placenta. The placenta is the connection between mother and baby, crucial for maintaining the pregnancy, providing nutrients and oxygen to the foetus, and removing waste material.

Men also need to consider that their sperm carry a lot of instructional information as well as genetic code. This information is located in the sperm head—kind of like its brain. It is this information that will determine whether the sperm can penetrate the ovum and whether cell division occurs properly, as well as affecting egg implantation and the integrity of the placenta. These are all vital components of conception. However, the sperm head is relatively unprotected and susceptible to oxidative damage.[3] When you consider that the instructions for early cell division and implantation rely on healthy sperm, giving them every possible protection becomes a very important consideration, especially when 50 per cent of miscarriages are linked to sperm malfunction.

During my time in clinic, it has been predominantly women who come in wanting to prepare for conception and pregnancy. The man rarely comes along to this very important discussion. Comments often given by the men include, "My mate smokes and drinks, and he had a healthy kid," or, "My swimmers are fine." Sorry, guys, this is not necessarily the case. Sperm are very delicate and highly susceptible to oxidative damage, which may render them less capable of successful fertilisation. I believe this lack of concern on the part of many men is mainly the result of insufficient awareness resulting from a strong focus on women when it comes to conception and pregnancy.

The four most crucial impacts on sperm quality are smoking, alcohol, radiation, and toxins.[4] Ejaculated sperm can vary in age from a few days to up to sixty days—the higher the age of sperm, the greater the exposure to oxidative damage. This type of damage can be caused by lifestyle factors such as smoking, consuming alcohol, sexually transmitted infections (STIs) and viral infections, obesity, pollution, industrial agents such as benzene, medications, toxins, and increasing age (which for men is thirty-five years and over). Viral infections not only impact sperm quality but can also be passed on during conception, infecting the foetus prior to birth. According to the World Health Organisation, common viruses implicated here include EBV, CMV, and all the human herpes group, which can lead to neonatal or childhood cancers.

Sperm are more vulnerable to toxic exposure and nutritional deficiency than are women's eggs. Sperm are generated consistently and are, therefore, exposed to any physiological or environmental hazards present at the time of generation. Sperm are also much smaller than eggs and are held outside the body, increasing their susceptibility, especially to physical trauma and heat.

Issues with sperm health can vary from poor sperm count to poor motility (movement), poor morphology (shape), and fragmented sperm DNA. When I used to look at sperm under the microscope, they tended to fall into one of three categories—the Olympic swimming champion, the spinner going around in circles, and the duds that just sat still and didn't move. Then there were the ones that looked healthy but had empty heads (damaged DNA or lacking in essential communication, preventing proper fertilisation and placental formation), which can't be identified under the microscope and requires special pathology assessment.

If you'd like to have your semen checked, speak to your GP for a referral to an andrology laboratory or fertility clinic—refer to Appendix 3 for laboratory details. To check motility, morphology, and volume, a semen analysis is carried out. However, to assess any DNA fragmentation a sperm chromatin structure assay (SCSA) will be required.

Francesca Naish from Natural Fertility Management,[5] writes, "While one in six couples is infertile, in 40 percent of cases the problem rests with the male, in 40 percent with the female, ten percent with both partners, and in a further ten percent of cases, the cause is unknown. Further, one in 25 males has a low sperm count and one in 35 is sterile."[6] These statistics highlight just how important it is that men take a more active role in preparing for a baby. The optimal time frame for preconception preparation is twelve months (I hear you gasp), but six months will also go a long way to increasing your chances of having a healthy baby. Your investment will depend on how committed you are in having a healthy baby.

There are many factors involved in the production of healthy sperm, and by addressing and supporting these, male fertility can be improved. The quality of seminal fluid—the fluid that bathes and protects the sperm on their journey towards the egg—is also important and has its own microbiome and specific pH (alkaline). The composition and pH of the semen interact with the woman's microbiome, strongly influencing fertility outcomes. Then there are the mitochondria—the energy producers that propel the sperm but also provide communication for fusion with the egg. It can take sperm two days to reach the egg, travelling a distance equivalent to an interstate trip, so you can begin to appreciate just how much energy is needed. Once the sperm arrive, they need to bind to the outer layer of the egg, penetrate, adhere, and fuse with the internal lining of the egg and block other sperm from entering; only then can the stages of cell division begin.

Whilst there are many herbs and nutritional supplements that can support male fertility, there are a few key nutrients that cannot be overlooked—zinc, selenium, and ubiquinol, or CoQ10. Nutritionally, zinc is of paramount importance for all sperm parameters and has been shown to increase count, motility, and morphology, as well as overall fertility.[7] Zinc deficiency is associated with reduced sperm numbers and testosterone levels, and men with normal sperm concentration have higher levels of zinc than those with reduced numbers.[8] Zinc supplementation has also been shown to reduce the incidence of anti-sperm antibodies in semen.[9]

In addition to zinc, healthy semen is also rich in selenium, which is an essential source of antioxidant protection against free radical damage. Oxidative stress is devastating to all sperm parameters, including DNA fragmentation. Unfortunately, zinc and selenium are two of the most common mineral deficiencies in Australia and New Zealand, due to the ancient soils in these countries. There are other antioxidants that can help protect the sperm and mitochondria from damage. Selenium acts on Leydig cells, which produce testosterone, regulating the hormone's production, improving sperm quality, and helping to prevent DNA fragmentation.[10] Adequate selenium has been associated with reduced miscarriage risk.[11]

The enzyme CoQ10, which provides both ubiquinone and ubiquinol, plays an essential role in protecting the mitochondria, and research has shown that it's associated with improved sperm count, motility, ejaculate volume, density, and morphology.[12] Now, before you go out and buy any supplements, *please wait* until you have read the section on diet and nutrition. Not all supplements are created equal, and one topic I am particularly passionate about is *quality*—so please read on. Other essential nutrients include vitamins A, C, E, D, and B complex, essential fatty acids, glutathione, calcium, and other minerals. For food sources, refer to Appendix 2.

While there are certain nutritional supplements available that help to support healthy sperm quality, these need to be taken for at least six months to achieve improved sperm motility, sperm concentrations, and sperm volume, not to mention healthy "information" to help with the vitally important early cell division of the fertilised egg. The reason for this time frame is because sperm take up to three months to develop and mature. But it can take many more months to remove heavy metals and other chemicals from the body. Therefore, a period of at least six months is recommended for men to prepare their bodies (and their sperm) for conception, a viable pregnancy, and a healthy baby but longer if chelation is required.

Diets lacking in fresh fruit and vegetables may be contributing to elevated levels of oxidative stress. In addition to addressing nutritional deficiencies, correct supplementation may significantly improve a man's sperm viability. Oxidative damage caused by free radicals may impair the sperm's energy production pathways, disable other functions, and damage its DNA. The resulting low sperm count and/or quality impairs fertility and increases the risk of passing on genetic defects. I'll explain more about oxidative stress, free radicals, and the effects of these on cell health in section III.

Male infertility is on the rise

Fertility expert Professor Peter Koopman at the University of Queensland says, "Since the 1970s, we have seen a huge increase in prevalence of male infertility and testicular cancer; this increase is directly attributable to environmental factors such as pollutants, cigarette smoke and exposure to chemicals."[13] In 2017, research found that, between 1973 and 2011, there was an average decline in mean sperm concentration of 1.6 per cent per year, and an overall decline of 59.3 per cent. A follow-up of the 2017 research revealed that sperm count is declining at an accelerated pace— 2.64 per cent after 2000 and an overall fall of 62.3 per cent, representing an overall decline of approximately 4.70 million sperm per year.[14] Obesity is also playing a key role, and this research showed that, with each five-kilogram increase in weight, there is a 5 per cent decline in sperm numbers and increase in DNA damage.

How best to deal with these environmentally destructive effects on sperm

When a cell is affected by oxidative stress, the resultant damage is likely to affect every part of it. This can include all the cell's critical functions including the energy-generating mitochondria, the protective membranes, key enzymes, and the DNA within the genes. Prevention is always better than treatment, so avoiding as many toxins as possible is highly advisable. You can read more about some of the most potent environmental toxins later in this section, but ensuring your body has good levels of antioxidants is essential.

One of the most powerful antioxidants in the body is superoxide dismutase (SOD), which protects sperm as they mature. Helping the body to regulate the antioxidants required has been shown to be a far more effective approach, rather than randomly taking high doses of vitamins. The best way to achieve this is to adopt a nutrigenomic strategy to support the body's own cellular defences. See the topic of diet and epigenetics for a more detailed discussion of nutrigenomics.[15] The power of SOD is such that it can extinguish between four and six million damaging free radical molecules per minute! Compare this with the effect of other more well-known antioxidants such as vitamins C and E and polyphenols such as grape seed and green tea, which extinguish just one free radical per molecule!

How lifestyle impacts male fertility

Lifestyle factors, especially those things you do daily or on a regular basis, have a huge impact on male reproductive health. Here are just a few of the most common:

- Smoking. Sperm concentrations in male smokers are 13 to 17 per cent lower than those in non-smokers, and cigarette smoking affects all sperm parameters, as well as lowering testosterone.
- Chronic alcohol intake affects male hormones by lowering testosterone and raising oestrogen, has a detrimental effect on semen quality and quantity, and raises inflammatory markers.
- Cannabis, opioids, and anabolic steroids lower testosterone and decrease sperm concentration, motility, and function. The effects of medicinal CBD oil on sperm quality are still being assessed.
- Caffeine at high levels lowers testosterone and sperm volume (this includes soft drinks, energy drinks, and some sports drinks).
- Advanced paternal age (APA) begins at age thirty-five in males, with an age-related decline in semen volume, normal sperm morphology, and sperm count and an increase in DNA fragmentation. APA is associated with lower pregnancy rates, miscarriage, and birth defects in the baby.
- General heat stress. Cycling as a sport has a strong association with increased testicular heat and subsequent oxidative stress. A study of male road cyclists found suppressed sperm parameters after a sixteen-week trial. Heat stress can also result from tight synthetic clothing or taking hot baths and saunas.
- Unhealthy diets consisting mainly of processed foods, such as cereals, breads, processed or deli meat, dairy, alcohol, coffee, soft drinks, fast foods, and low fresh fruit and vegetable intake are associated with poor semen quality and lower fertility rates.

- Insufficient sleep of less than six hours per day lowers sperm motility and contributes to DNA damage.[16]
- Exposure to electromagnetic frequencies (EMF) may alter both DNA and cellular integrity, as well as causing heat stress. Keep all electronic equipment such as laptops, mobile phones, and tablets well away from your lap.[17]
- Environmental chemicals, including herbicides, pesticides, petrochemicals, paints, solvents, and lots more, can impact sperm as you'll see in chapter 4, "Environmental Toxins."

It's all about the nutrients

The good news is that there is clinical evidence that several herbs, as well as good nutrition can help to improve fertility in men. A sperm's structure is basically made of nutrients, which means it can be positively influenced by good diet and antioxidants. Nutrients and foods that provide these are listed in Appendix 2. Remember, it takes three months for sperm to develop. Keep this in mind when deciding to start a family, as you will need to support your system for at least three months, but preferably six to twelve months, if you are seeking to father a healthy baby. Every chemical you can avoid is one less toxin for your body to deal with. If you have been exposed to a number of chemicals or have a high heavy metal load in your body, you may need to allocate at least twelve months to properly clear these toxins from your body before considering having a baby.

Food is our body's source of nutrients, so it is important that you select only organic, unsprayed produce and animal products that come from unsprayed pasture-fed farms.

Another common source of toxins is work-related chemical exposure. So *always* wear protective clothing and equipment. The Australian adage of, "She'll be right, mate," and taking the "tough bloke" stance won't protect your sperm from toxin damage. Wear the protective mask, gloves, and whatever protective clothing is implicated in any work you do— whether on the job or around the home.

***

- ❖ The four most crucial impacts on sperm quality are smoking, alcohol, radiation, and toxins.[18]
- ❖ A full 40 per cent of miscarriage cases are the result of poor sperm quality.
- ❖ Insufficient sleep of less than six hours per day lowers sperm motility and contributes to DNA damage.
- ❖ Exposure to electromagnetic frequencies (EMF) may alter both DNA and cellular integrity, in addition to causing heat stress. Keep all electronic equipment such as laptops, mobile phones, and tablets well away from your lap.

2

Your Turn, Ladies

In the twenty-first century, there is a growing trend to postpone conception well into the thirties and even forties, whereas, previously, most couples were starting families in their twenties. This delay in childbirth is just one piece of the infertility puzzle, with other lifestyle, environmental, and genetic aspects contributing to reduced fertility.

Lifestyle factors that have a detrimental effect on reproduction are predominantly linked to the rising rates of obesity, with two out of three Australian adults now overweight or obese. However, factors such as excessive exercise; low peripheral body fat; smoking; drug use (recreational as well as pharmaceutical drugs, including the birth control pill, implants, or injections); genetically modified foods; exposure to toxic chemicals; and sexually-transmitted diseases are all lifestyle contributors to female infertility.

The four most critical factors influencing women's fertility are diet, drugs, smoking, and alcohol.[19] There is nothing positive about smoking for egg health; indeed, it causes increased follicle loss. Even sleeping next to a partner or being exposed to semen from a smoker has a negative correlation to the female microbiome, egg quality, and overall fertility.

There is a significant difference between how toxins affect the gonads of men and women. Whereas men's gonads don't begin making sperm until puberty, women are born with their lifetime supply of eggs (oocytes). "A female fetus produces all of her eggs very early in the gestational cycle. During the time when those eggs are being produced, they are extremely sensitive to environmental insults."[20] Dr Seneff goes on to say that female foetuses exposed to environmental toxins while in utero can experience genetic mutations and epigenetic effects that may be passed on through multiple future generations.[21] In other words, exposure of the mother to chemicals and toxins during pregnancy affects the quality of the unborn daughter's oocytes. This fact alone really highlights the long-term effects that exposure to toxins during pregnancy can have, not only on your unborn baby but also on future generations.

Most of the same lifestyle factors impacting male reproductive health also affect women—smoking, alcohol, diet, radiation, and the myriad of environmental toxins we are exposed to daily. And it is these toxins and lifestyle factors that also affect the health of a woman's uterus and reproductive capacity. Obesity in women is a huge factor, as the fat cells, known as adipose tissue, produce hormones themselves, as well as pro-inflammatory substances and toxins. Obesity is also linked with inferior quality of oocytes, increasing chromosomal damage and DNA abnormality. There is also an increased risk of miscarriage with excess weight, as well as other metabolic-related conditions.

Rising rates of conditions such as PCOS, endometriosis, and uterine fibroids all represent further challenges to fertility, alongside genetic influences that can limit or decrease ovarian reserve (the total number of oocytes within the ovary). PCOS is one of the most common causes of female infertility and endocrine disorders in women and is associated with metabolic conditions such as obesity, insulin resistance, and increased risk of developing type 2 diabetes and cardiovascular disease. Women with PCOS also have a higher risk of having children with autism.[22]

While endometriosis has been grossly underdiagnosed, awareness in the medical field is improving, and research is providing more answers—relating not only to contributing factors but also to support. These are specialised areas that require individual assessment and care. So please, if you suspect or have been diagnosed with PCOS or endometriosis or experience any menstrual pain, consult a qualified health practitioner; also consider seeing a naturopath. Your monthly cycle should not be painful, extensive, or debilitating. From my experience in clinic, many factors can be positively influenced to make the monthly cycle pain-free, regular, and asymptomatic.

Microbes, inflammation, and sleep

It is essential that any residual viral infections be totally cleared from your body prior to conception to avoid infecting the foetus. Partners generally share and reinfect each other with viruses, so both of you need to be assessed for the presence of any infection and treated accordingly well before trying to have a baby.

As viruses live inside our cells, they can be difficult to treat, with medications often causing problems of their own. The most effective method I have found—and have used extensively in clinic for many years—is frequency therapy. Using specific frequencies to clear viruses and other non-beneficial microbes from the body is not only safe but also highly effective, as the waves can pass through healthy cells and tissue, only affecting the microbes being targeted. While there are many people advertising various forms of frequency therapy, it is important to ensure they are properly qualified natural medicine practitioners, as opposed to just having done a quick online course or, worse, no training at all.

You also have the option of investing in a device to use at home—this is my preferred option, as you then have a device you can use for many years to come, which is particularly helpful when you have children. Appendix 4 lists my preferred suppliers.

On hearing the term "microbiome," most people think about the gut. That would be correct. But did you know that you also have specific strains that live in your vagina, cervix, uterus lining, and fallopian tubes? These microbes directly affect conception. But it gets better—the interaction between the woman's vaginal microbiome with the microbiome of the man's semen affects the gender of the sperm. Further up the reproductive tract, the microbiome affects sperm binding with the oocyte.[23] If you thought you only had microbes in your gut, please know you have them in your reproductive organs as well. While gut health affects your reproductive microbes, oral health affects the placenta. Just another reason to ensure your digestive health is optimal well prior to conception.

Excessive and vigorous exercise can disrupt ovulation in women with normal body mass or weight. However, moderate exercise has shown to be highly beneficial in restoring ovulation in obese women with ovulatory disorders like PCOS. Excessive exercise is also a source of inflammation and oxidative stress, often resulting in low pH (tissue acidity). Therefore, it is advisable to keep exercise and movement within your fitness levels. And if you are starting out on your exercise journey, remember to take it slowly and gradually build up duration and intensity. Going hard or going home is not always the safest approach.

Sleep is also essential for good fertility, as there is a negative relationship between insufficient / poor quality sleep and human growth hormone.[24]

Another hormone that can be greatly influenced by lifestyle is anti-müllerian hormone (AMH). Binging on alcoholic drinks twice or more a week can lower AMH by 26 per cent.[25] AMH levels directly correlate with fertility outcomes. All these lifestyle factors affect the integrity of the woman's eggs, which perform some amazing tasks. One fact that particularly blew me away is that, when the male sperm enters the ovum, she checks him out. If he is damaged in any way, she works her magic to repair that damage before enabling coupling and cell division. This repair of damaged sperm DNA helps prevent passing on polymorphisms to the baby. However, if the oocyte is tired as a result of high toxic load, she cannot manage to correct any sperm deficiencies. Our bodies, given the right support, are nothing short of amazing!

Avoiding future complications

While I will go into much more detail about nutrition in section II, I would like to stress that the same advice applies to the preparation phase —and remember that preparation includes clearing your body of all toxins, so this period can cover many months. Nutrients are essential for your body to do its job, which also encompasses the clearance of toxins, as well as repairing any damage these toxins may have caused. Good nutrition is essential for all stages of motherhood, and the earlier you adopt healthy habits around food and lifestyle, the easier it becomes. All the information outlined in section II, as well as food sources listed in Appendix 2, apply to the preparation phase just as much as during pregnancy.

If you have been experiencing difficulties in conceiving, the pathology tests suggested in Appendix 3 may help shed light on possible causes. Here's just one example of why tests can be helpful— elevated free copper can stop you from conceiving, as high copper causes the body to think it is pregnant. Simply by removing the excess copper, conception may occur faster than you think.

I will explain more about the impacts of how everything you do affects the developing foetus and baby in sections II and III—but there is absolutely no reason not to take these recommendations on board as soon as you decide you would one day like to start a family. Thorough preparation sets a solid foundation, which you will appreciate more when you understand what happens inside you once fertilisation has occurred. Every woman carries the genetic blueprint her grandchildren will inherit, giving women the power to ensure that future generations will inherit the very best genetic information possible.

In addition to conception issues, complications during pregnancy are also on the increase and can include high blood pressure, heart problems, obesity, postpartum haemorrhage, or premature births. The United States has the highest rate of death on the first day of life among industrialised nations.[26] Extensive evidence has suggested that environmental factors such as phthalate, glyphosate, dioxin, and bisphenol A exposure have significant links with conditions such as endometriosis and ovarian reserve, as well as gonadal damage, oocyte development and maturation. Environmental toxins have a huge impact on your unborn baby's health and, according to environmental specialist Dr Mark Donohoe, "greatly affect behavioural problems and autism."[27]

Healthy teeth and gums

One aspect that may be overlooked during the preparation phase is oral health. Ensure that you have seen your dentist and corrected any oral health issues well before trying to start a family.[28] This includes removing any old amalgam (silver) fillings, as these have been shown to leach mercury into the body, which will affect the baby growing inside you. For example, mercury has been linked to the development of cleft pallet in the developing foetus. Mercury is a toxic heavy metal that accumulates in tissues, including kidneys, eyes, brain, thyroid, and liver—definitely not recommended for a developing foetus. Therefore, removal, followed by supervised detoxification, is one of the first things to tick off your preparation list.

Furthermore, ensuring healthy gums and a healthy oral microbiome are important preventative measures against any possible decay forming during pregnancy when repair work and materials used may affect your unborn baby.

Perhaps a lesser known fact is that a mother's dental or oral health determines the placental microbiome. Whereas the mother's digestive or gut microbiome influences the uterine environment. Therefore, it is essential that the mother ensures both oral and digestive health are optimal to avoid things that could negatively interfere with the environment the baby is growing in. The microbiome will shape the health and immunity of that child, while also influencing implantation and miscarriage. Factors that affect the mother's microbiome include exposure to toxins, environmental pollutants, poor dietary choices, stress, and her partner's microbiome—topics that are discussed in greater detail in the coming chapters.

Men and women's roles are different but equally important. Whether you are having the baby yourself or using egg or sperm donors or a surrogate, each person involved should heed the above advice to give the baby the very best opportunity for a healthy and long life.

***

- ❖ The four most critical factors influencing women's fertility are diet, drugs, smoking, and alcohol.
- ❖ Your role as mother-to-be requires diligent preparation, including a healthy diet and lifestyle.
- ❖ Aim for a minimum of eight hours sleep every night.
- ❖ Seek qualified advice, individual assessment, and tailored support.

3

Sperm Meets Egg

> Life is the division of human cells, a process which begins at conception.
>
> —Dick Gephardt

What happens when sperm meets egg?

In order for you to fully appreciate the magnitude of creating a new life, I'd like to go into a little biology. I'll try and keep it simple. But for those who prefer to learn more, I have included a few links at the end of this chapter. Understanding the following paragraphs should strengthen your commitment to making every effort to prepare for conception. Once the egg is fertilised, the creation of a new life is locked in to a set timeline. The development of the foetus relies on specific nutrients being available in the correct quantities at the correct time—if one single nutrient is not available at the time an organ is being formed, then that organ may be damaged, impaired, or not function properly.

When a healthy sperm meets the egg, it fuses with the ovum, creating a protective layer preventing any other sperm from also entering. The instructions in the sperm head trigger the process of cell division. One cell becomes two, two become four, four become eight, and so forth. This ball of rapidly dividing cells is called the blastocyst, which embeds into the uterus wall around day nine. From this early stage, the first of three embryonic or primordial tissues begins to form.

The three primordial or embryonic tissues are the endoderm, the ectoderm, and the mesoderm. Don't get hung up on the names, which may sound quite strange. Think of them as the foundation of a house—footings, concrete, and walls giving rise to rooms, plumbing, electrical wiring, windows, ceilings, and doors. Each foundational element must be sound, or the building may develop cracks or even crumble. The same principle applies when creating a baby—each step must be completed correctly on a set day of development. Remember this sentence: **Every**

stage of development must occur in sequence—if a building block (nutrient) is missing, that moment's development remains incomplete. The first of the primordial tissues to form is the endoderm, which goes on to become parts of the digestive tract, ear, respiratory tract, and bladder, as well as prostate and lower vagina. By week three, all embryonic tissues are getting into full swing, creating the different parts of a body that will become a foetus and, after about nine months, a baby. These phases are outlined more fully in table 1, which shows the timeline of tissue development.[29] Consider that the central nervous system, including the spinal column, begins to form on day eighteen after fertilisation—a vital component of the body is forming well before the woman may even realise she is pregnant.

Throughout the entire gestation period, cells divide and turn into specific tissues and organs based on the three embryonic tissues mentioned above. The time of differentiation of each and every cell follows a set time frame—there is no deviation and no room for error or compromise.

In order for a specific tissue to be created, certain nutrients must be present and available. These nutrients include amino acids, vitamins, minerals, and fats. For example, if one single nutrient is not available on any day that heart tissue is being formed, then the heart may not develop correctly. There's no going back. The embryonic period does not allow for missing nutrients or building blocks; nor does it go back and repair once that nutrient is available. This is why it is so very important that the mum-to-be's nutritional status is optimal well prior to conception and throughout pregnancy.

Table 1. Primordial tissues

Endoderm

- Epithelium of the gastrointestinal tract, except its terminal parts, and the parenchyma of glands derived from it (liver, pancreas, thyroid, parathyroid, thymus)
- Lining epithelium of the eustachian tube and of middle ear cavity, including inner layer of eardrum and lining of the mastoid air cells
- Lining epithelium of the respiratory tract—larynx, trachea, bronchi, alveoli
- Epithelium of the bladder, most of the female urethra and part of the male urethra, plus the glands derived from them (prostate), lower part of the vagina

Ectoderm

- Skin and its appendages—epithelium of skin, hair, and nails and epithelial cells of sweat, sebaceous glands, and mammary glands
- Epithelium of the beginning and end of the gastrointestinal tract—epithelium and glands, cheeks, gums, part of the floor of the mouth and palate, and mucous membranes of the nasal cavities and paranasal sinuses, as well as epithelium of the lower part of the anal canal and terminal parts of the genital and urinary tracts
- Tissues of the nervous system (entire CNS), including retina, peripheral nervous system including sympathetic nerve cells and fibres, the medulla of the adrenal gland and neurilemmal sheath cells, and the sensory epithelium of the olfactory and auditory organs
- Anterior pituitary
- Lens of the eye, anterior epithelial layer of the cornea, muscles of the iris, optic nerve, and outer layer of the eardrum

Mesoderm

- Visceral and parietal linings of the peritoneal, pleural, and pericardial cavities
- Cortex of adrenal gland (stress affects this tissue type)
- Connective tissue, cartilage, and bone, including dentine; myocardium and visceral musculature, including blood vessels, endocardium, and endothelium of blood vessels
- Lymph glands, lymph vessels, and spleen
- Blood cells
- Connective tissue sheaths of muscles, tendons, and nerve endings; the synovial membranes of joints and bursae

Just consider the number of tissues formed during the first three weeks of pregnancy, a time when most women are not even aware of what's happening inside them. And it's not only nutrients that play a pivotal role in the health of the developing tissues but also toxins that may be present. Toxins act like a block to production. For example, the upper mouth and pallet form during week three as part of the ectoderm. If elevated levels of mercury are present, cleft pallet may result.

Indeed, if nutrients are missing or deficient or toxins block production in any of the three primordial tissues, all related organs will be affected. As an example, let's consider ear problems. Ears are part of the endoderm. So, if a baby has chronic ear problems, then other endoderm-related tissues may also have been affected during formation.

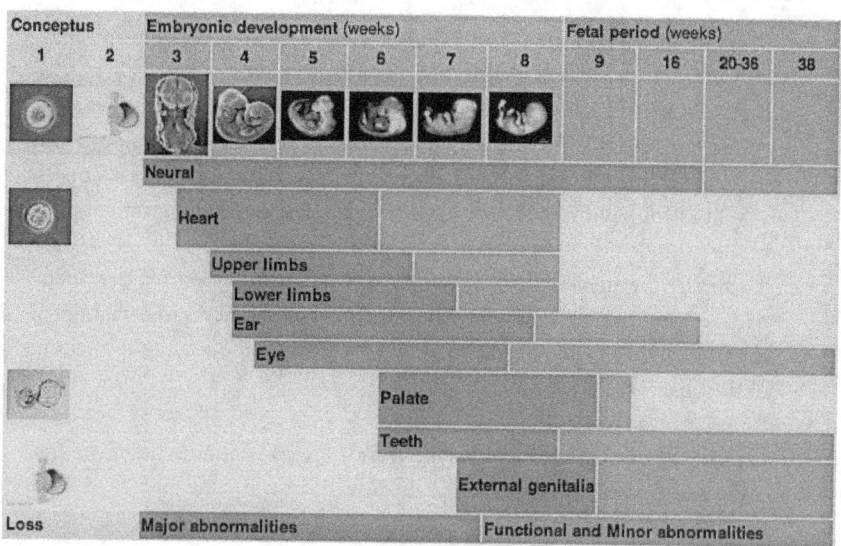

Table 2. Timeline showing development of your baby from conception to birth[30]

***

For a comprehensive outline of what is happening throughout gestation, visit a website called Embryology, dedicated to education and research on the subject. You can find it online at https://embryology.med.unsw.edu.au/embryology/index.php/Main_Page.

For an example of how any problems in one of the three primordial tissues can affect related organs refer to:
https://pubmed.ncbi.nlm.nih.gov/33308219/.

***

- ❖ Every nutrient must be available throughout the entire gestation period—no exceptions.
- ❖ Avoid chemicals and toxins—ensure proper detoxification is completed well prior to conception.
- ❖ Provide the safest possible environment for your baby to grow in.

4

Environmental Toxins

> Americans of all ages are carrying around over 219 toxic chemicals in their body at any given time.
> —Center for Disease Control 2009, *Fourth National Report on Human Exposure to Chemicals*

It's time to take a closer look at all the environmental toxins we're exposed to in our modern lives. This is *huge*, as most people are unaware of just how many chemicals and toxins we are exposed to every single day. I have dedicated a lot of book space to the topic of toxins and how they impact your body and, more particularly, the unborn and newly born baby. The following information is not intended to create stress but, rather, awareness and understanding.

After explaining the extent of chemicals in our environment, I'll introduce you to some of those more commonly used throughout the world. Then I'll explain how you can identify and reduce your exposure, as well as testing options and tips on how to clear any toxic substances from your body. I've only touched on the basics, but if this piques your interest and you want to learn more, there is a list of recommended reading at the end of the book. So please do take the time to read through it all—you can read it in stages, that's perfectly OK. Many references are provided throughout the following text should you like to research this important issue in greater depth.

The Chemical Abstract Service notes that, in 1954, some six hundred thousand chemical compounds had been synthesised and documented;[31] at the end of 1993, the media reported that a Japanese research team had synthesised the twelve millionth chemical compound; and by 2009, the number had increased to fifty million. In the United States alone, a new chemical is synthesised every minute. Most of these were unknown just two generations ago.

In terms of amounts, 400 million tonnes are produced annually, with about half of the chemicals in use having annual production levels exceeding 500,000 kilograms. Each year, 4.5 billion litres of pesticides are sprayed on crops in Britain alone. Take a moment to digest these figures. They can be quite overwhelming. Is it any wonder we as a human race are becoming increasingly health challenged?

Chemicals can enter our bodies in one of three ways and can cause inflammation either by direct contact or indirectly by stimulating an immune response:

- ingestion in food or water,
- inhalation, or
- skin contact.

When the term "environmental toxins" is used, we tend not to associate these with our immediate surroundings. It has been said that the environment inside the home can be more polluted than outside. Toxins inside the home include formaldehyde from fabrics, carpets, furniture, and bedding; plastics; car fumes from garages; cooking gas (which is particularly implicated in asthma); pine furniture; cleaning products and bleaches; glues in furnishings and cabinetry; home office products (printing toners); air fresheners and perfumes; and antimony from clothing and drinking bottles, as well as medications. When inhaled in sufficient doses, chemical exposure contributes to asthma.

Environmental health research has identified the presence of numerous toxic chemicals in pregnant women. Many of the chemicals found have been banned since the 1970s but are still abundantly present in our environment. This is because many chemicals just do not break down but, instead, remain in soil and water for many decades after being used. For this reason, it is imperative to ensure your body is free of chemicals and heavy metals prior to conceiving a child. This applies to both parents—not only the mother.

In the United States, researchers analysing data for more than 160 chemicals detected polychlorinated biphenyls (PCBs), organochlorine pesticides, perfluorinated compounds (PFCs), phenols, polybrominated diphenyl ethers (PBDEs), phthalates, polycyclic aromatic hydrocarbons (PAHs) and perchlorate in 99 to 100 per cent of pregnant women. On January

16, 2011, ScienceDaily reported, "Among the chemicals found in the study group were PBDEs, compounds used as flame retardants now banned in many states including California, and dichlorodiphenyltrichloroethane (DDT), an organochlorine pesticide banned in the United States in 1972." Chemicals are manufactured and used by industries worldwide. These chemicals enter our food, water, air, personal care products, and direct environments, including our homes and workplaces. Toxins are everywhere, and we are all exposed. You can't avoid them all, but you can take steps to avoid as many toxic chemicals as possible.

Never is this more important than prior to conception and throughout pregnancy. The placenta concentrates heavy metals and toxic substances only to have them enter the innocent unborn. During the formation of the foetus, there are what is known as critical windows of development of primordial tissues, discussed previously. This relates to the development of certain tissue that, when disturbed by toxins or lack of nutrients, will never form properly, resulting in permanent damage.

How environmental toxins affect the unborn

A baby's exposure to toxic compounds while in the uterus may cause cancer or make the child more susceptible to cancer and other diseases later in life. Many of these chemicals also damage other body systems that can impact development, reproduction, brain function, immune health, and more. Chronic childhood diseases linked to toxic chemical exposure have been surging upward for years, and experts believe rising rates of birth defects, asthma, neurodevelopmental disorders, and other serious diseases in US children are a result of early chemical exposure.

It is also directly a result of the mother's chemical load that newborn babies are being born toxic. One study by the Environmental Working Group (EWG) found that blood samples from newborns contained an average of 287 toxins, including mercury, fire retardants, pesticides, and Teflon chemicals. Evidence suggests that prenatal and early life exposure to environmental persistent organic pollutants (POPs), including herbicides, pesticides, cigarette smoke, heavy metals, and certain medications, play a role in foetal programming and are contributing to the current obesity epidemic. In other words, **what your baby is exposed to while in utero** will have a major impact on its health later in life and possibly on future generations as well.

The term "obesogen" has been coined to describe substances that disrupt normal fat metabolism. As the exact extent of these obesogens is not yet fully known, it is recommended that pregnant and breastfeeding women avoid all toxins wherever possible. All too often, we're not even aware of exposure to toxic substances. So, it's highly recommended that both parents be assessed for mineral imbalances and presence of toxins well prior to conception, as it can take up to eighteen months to fully remove some heavy metals from the body. A very easy way to check some of these is with a hair tissue mineral analysis or HTMA (details in Appendix 3). You can also do a quick review of how toxic your body is from the list of common products in the section that follows.

Surrounded by chemicals

"It is estimated that by 2050, two billion tonnes of chemical additives will have been used in plastic."[32] Many of the chemicals in plastic are toxic and leach into the environment during manufacturing, use, and disposal. Don't be lulled into a sense of security by using compostable plastics, as these break down into nano or microparticles, which enter the life cycle of all living organisms—and that includes humans. Microplastics have been shown to correlate with AMH deficiency, affecting the health of oocytes, as well as having a direct negative correlation with all fertility parameters.[33] Two chemicals used in the manufacturing of plastic that are of global concern are BPA and phthalates (pronounced /falates/). BPA is an oestrogenic environmental toxin with potentially serious effects on human health. It is classified as the third most important pollutant and an endocrine (hormone) disrupter. What's concerning is that we have known BPA has oestrogenic effects since the early 1930s. Recent studies have confirmed it to be a known endocrine disruptor, associated with reproductive disorders, breast cancer, obesity, neurological disorders, and cardiovascular disease.

Chemicals are virtually everywhere in the modern world, lurking in personal care products, food containers, medical tubing, toys, and more.

Some of the top offenders you should be aware of, and watch out for, include:

- **Phthalates.** Exposure to phthalates can lead to incomplete testicular descent in foetuses, reduced sperm counts in men, and testicular atrophy or structural abnormality and inflammation in newborns.[34] The effects of this chemical involve fertility and the child but can also extend three to four generations in the future.[35] Phthalates are found in vinyl flooring, detergents, automotive plastics, soap, shampoo, deodorants, fragrances, hair-spray, nail polish, plastic bags, food packaging, garden hoses, inflatable toys, blood-storage bags, and intravenous medical tubing.

- **Bisphenol A (BPA).** A common ingredient in many plastics—including reusable water bottles and resins lining some food cans and take-away coffee cups, dental sealants, toys, receipt paper, and plumbing water pipes—BPA can change the course of foetal development, as well as increase risk of miscarriage and breast cancer. Polycarbonate plastics contain BPA. BPA has been detected in the umbilical cord blood of 90 per cent of newborn infants tested.[36] Always check the base of plastic containers for a BPA-free imprint.

- **Microplastics.** When plastics break down into particles less than five millimetres in size, they are termed "microplastics." These microparticles move through the environment in soil and water and are easily absorbed by all living organisms—plants, fish, and other animals—to end up in our bloodstream. Scientists have found small plastic fragments in the human placenta.[37] Microplastics affect human health across our lifespan, contributing to[38]
    - endocrine disruption, which leads to cancer (breast, prostate, testes), cardiovascular disease, metabolic disorders (obesity, diabetes), reproductive issues (genital malformations, infertility, early puberty, foetal damage);
    - neurodevelopment and, thus, learning disorders, and autism spectrum disorders;[39]

- immune system activation, leading to asthma and autoimmune disease;
- reduced foetal growth;
- pre-eclampsia; and
- DNA or chromosomal damage.

- **Perfluorooctanoic acid (PFOA).** Found in grease and water-resistant coatings like Teflon and Gore-Tex, PFOA is considered a likely carcinogen.[40]

- **Methoxychlor and vinclozin.** An insecticide and a fungicide respectively, methoxychlor and vinclozin have been found to cause changes to male mice born for as many as four subsequent generations after the initial exposure. In humans, it has been identified as impacting male fertility and altering genes.[41]

- **Nonylphenol ethoxylates (NPEs).** NPEs are known to be potent endocrine disrupters.[42] These chemicals are found in laundry detergents, personal hygiene products, automotive and latex paints, and lawn care products. They turn certain genes on or off, which interferes with the way your glandular system works. They mimic the female hormone oestrogen and have been implicated as one reason behind some marine species switching from male to female.

- **Bovine growth hormones** commonly added to commercial dairy cows have been implicated as a contributor to premature adolescence.

- **Non-fermented and GMO soy products** contain hormone-like substances and glyphosate, which is known to disrupt our gut microbiome and act as an endocrine disrupter. Glyphosate is sprayed on GMO crops and is a major offender on the toxin list—so much so it requires an entire book for itself. I highly recommend you read Dr Stephanie Seneff's *Toxic Legacy: How the Weedkiller Glyphosate Is Destroying Our Health and the Environment.*

- **MSG.** A food additive and flavour enhancer widely used in some Asian cuisines and processed foods, MSG has been linked to reduced fertility and neurological disorders, including depression.[43]

- **Fluoride.** This chemical in our water supply has been linked to lower fertility rates, hormone disruption, and low sperm counts, as well as possibly toxic to the developing brain.[44] This is why it's highly recommended not to use regular tap water when preparing any baby formula or foods. There is some confusion as to the difference between naturally occurring calcium fluoride (which is beneficial for bones and teeth) and industrialised forms that are added to water supplies in Australia and North America. There are three types of fluoride used to fluoridate water supplies—fluorosilicic acid, sodium fluorosilicate, and sodium fluoride. Fluorosilicic acid is the type most often used for cost reasons, and it is derived from phosphate fertilisers and, given what we know about the dangers of these, you may now understand why I recommend investing in a good water filter to ensure fluoride is removed from the water you and your family consume.

What each of these substances has in common is that they can affect your and your children's endocrine system and reproductive health. The action of these and other substances in our environment and on our genes is called epigenetics, which will be explained later.

The glands of your endocrine system and the hormones they release influence nearly every cell, organ, and function of your body. Hormones are messengers, instrumental in regulating mood, growth and development, tissue function, and metabolism, as well as sexual function and reproductive processes. Numerous studies over the past decade confirm that males may be particularly at risk to the chemicals listed above. Decreased sperm motility and concentration, as well as genital abnormalities in baby boys have been linked to these chemicals.

Endocrine-disrupting chemicals

The more a pregnant woman is exposed to high levels of the endocrine-disrupter known as phthalates, the greater the risk her son will have smaller genitals and incomplete testicular descent, leading to impaired reproductive development. The chemical also appears to make the overall genital tracts of boys slightly more feminine. It is believed that phthalates have these adverse effects because they reduce testosterone synthesis by interfering with an enzyme needed to produce the male hormone.[45]

In one study, women who had higher concentrations of two types of phthalates (DEHP and DBP) also had boys who appeared more feminised in their personality while playing. The presence of phthalates in the mothers was not associated with any differences in the girls' play behaviour. However, that is not an indication that phthalates are safe for girls. Phthalates also affect women's endocrine systems and reproductive health although the effects are different between the genders. For instance, girls are reaching puberty earlier than ever before.[46] And these chemicals may be culprits.

Bovine growth hormones used in food production, non-fermented GMO soy foods, and bisphenol-A (BPA), just to name a few, add to the problem, as they also mimic oestrogen and disrupt the endocrine system. Endocrine-disrupting chemicals including DDT, bisphenol, resorcinol, and birth control pill hormones have all been found in waterways and recycled drinking water. Traditional waste-water treatment plants do not remove these drugs.[47] Other studies have linked the chemicals to thyroid problems in both women and men, and researchers have also suggested a link between phthalates and illnesses like allergies, asthma, and contact dermatitis, all of which are on the rise in children.

Thanks to more research and publication of findings, we now have access to where these chemicals are found, giving us the option to avoid affected products. This awareness has also seen a rise in chemical-free products for home, garden, and personal use—check the stores, read labels for ingredients, and take steps to avoid exposure to dangerous chemicals. A whole host of toxins will affect the unborn child throughout its life. These substances are also known as teratogens or drug-induced birth defects. The potential for drug-induced birth defects is significantly increased during early pregnancy, especially during the period of embryonic development, as this early phase of pregnancy may often go undetected. Therefore, every sexually active female should be aware of the possibility of pregnancy and associated risk of birth defects attributed to some substances. A 2004 study found that pregnant women are regularly taking an average of thirteen medications.[48] Commonly used drugs include alcohol, antibiotics, antacids, analgesics, antimicrobials, tranquilisers, and diuretics, supporting the call for a greater awareness of teratogenic actions of these and other substances, including recreational and illicit drugs.

Dangers of socially accepted drugs

Marketing strategies targeting fast relief from pain often result in the promiscuous use of these drugs. One only has to watch television briefly to be exposed to advertisers promoting pain relief. It is not only analgesics that give rise for concern. Adverse effects of alcohol consumption, as well as incorrect dosages or poor-quality supplements are often overlooked by the unknowing mother-to-be. In order to properly cater to the health and well-being of an unborn child, it is important to understand the mechanism of how commonly prescribed and over-the-counter substances consumed during pregnancy can cause birth defects.

- **Antibiotic and anticoagulant medication**
  Some antibiotic medications are able to cross the placental membrane and be deposited in the embryo's bones and teeth at sites of active calcification. As little as one gram per day of tetracycline administered during the third trimester of pregnancy can produce yellow staining of both primary and secondary teeth. When used from as early as the fourth month, it may cause tooth defects and diminished growth of long bones. Antibiotics including streptomycin and dihydrostreptomycin can damage the eighth cranial nerve, vestibulocochlear, causing deafness in infants whose mothers have been treated with high doses of these drugs.[49] Moore and Persaud further note that the popular anticoagulant warfarin is a definite teratogen following research carried out in Philadelphia, Pennsylvania, United States. They report on mothers who took this anticoagulant during the critical period of embryonic development (between weeks six and twelve) whose children suffered hypoplasia of the nasal cartilage, stippled epiphyses, and various central nervous system defects.

- **Analgesic, decongestant, andanti-inflammatory drugs**
Analgesics are readily available over the counter from the chemist, as well as the supermarket. As a result of easy access, the wide-ranging effects of analgesics are often forgotten and not put into context of being potentially dangerous to the defenceless unborn. Some of the more common non-steroidal anti-inflammatory drugs (NSAIDs) contain ibuprofen, acetylsalicylic acid (more commonly known as aspirin), and paracetamol (also known as acetaminophen). A study involving ingestion of ibuprofen during pregnancy found the substance disturbed embryonic implantation, inhibition of the birthing processes, and contraction of blood vessels leading to maternal pulmonary hypertension.[50] Gastroschisis is a congenital ibuprofen-related malformation in which foetal organs develop outside the abdominal wall. Other drug-related cases of gastroschisis have been linked to maternal use of other NSAIDs and the decongestants pseudoephedrine and phenylpropanolamine.[51]

Some analgesics enjoy a reputation of being generally safe to use during pregnancy except during the latter months due to the inhibition of hormones affecting birth. Despite being considered safe to use, acetylsalicylic acid, taken in high doses, as shown in a 2001 report involving human trials, may produce a variety of congenital malformations.[52] Due to the emotionally charged aspect of conducting human trials on pregnant women, results of research on animals including rats and rabbits provide much of the data. Use of NSAIDs during the first trimester of pregnancy in human trials were shown to cause ventricular septal defects, midline defects, diaphragmatic hernias, and hydrocephalus in the foetus.[53] Most defects occurred when administered during days six to seventeen following fertilisation—further highlighting the importance of early-stage pregnancy abstinence from drugs.

I also find it interesting that these conditions known to result from certain medications are often categorised as "congenital," inferring there is no known cause, when we know exactly when embryonic and foetal tissues are being formed.

- **Antiviral and antifungal medication**
 The antiviral group of drugs varies in its application, being used either topically or ingested, with duration of treatment depending on the specific condition involved. With the increase in viral herpes infections, including recurrent genital herpes, some medications prescribed for continuous administration have been linked with foetal structural malformations.[54] The link here is that medications prescribed to block viral reproduction alter DNA metabolism, particularly affecting those phases of rapid cell division of embryonic development, as well as throughout the entire pregnancy.

 Published trials of foetal defects attributed to virustatic agents include skull bone abnormalities such as malformation of the tympanic membrane, impaired immune function due to reduced thymus and increased spleen.[55]

 According to the Australian Food and Drug Administration (FDA), repeated doses of antifungal creams, used to treat vaginal thrush, have been associated with a "consistent pattern of birth defects"[56] similar to those seen in animal studies. Other reports involve trisomy, which is a chromosomal abnormality often seen in Down's syndrome.

- **Mood stabilisers, antidepressants, tranquilisers, and hypnotics**
 Although this category of drugs usually requires a prescription, it may often be taken for longer periods of time and commenced well before the woman conceives. The Australian Bureau of Statistics (2006) reports that more than sixteen thousand women aged between eighteen and forty-four years had taken antidepressant medication during the two weeks preceding the 2004-05 survey. It is acknowledged that benzodiazepines are the most commonly used drugs in the United States for the treatment of anxiety, phobias, and tension.[57] Human trials have revealed that diazepam, a benzodiazepine, passes into the placenta from week six of gestation, transferring the drug into both amniotic fluid and foetal tissues during organ development.[58]

The effects of taking benzodiazepine drugs during pregnancy may lead to foetal abortion, malformation, intrauterine growth retardation, functional deficits, carcinogenesis, and mutagenesis, with greatest risks occurring between two and eight weeks after conception. When the drug is used near term, foetal dependence and withdrawal have been known to occur.

A recent study conducted at the University of Montreal, Canada, revealed that taking more than twenty-five milligrams per day of paroxetine during the first trimester of pregnancy may cause major congenital and cardiac malformations.[59] Paroxetine is one of many selective serotonin reuptake inhibitors (SSRIs) frequently prescribed in cases of mild depression or anxiety. In 2005, the drug manufacturers GlaxoSmithKline and the American FDA warned of congenital malformations in infants born to women taking Paxil (brand name for paroxetine) (Consumer Affairs, 2005).

Another drug commonly prescribed as a mood stabiliser is the carboxamide carbamazepine. Although traditionally associated with the treatment of more severe psychiatric conditions, including bipolar disorder and schizophrenia; as an anticonvulsant; and for trigeminal neuralgia, carbamazepine has become widely used by many women coming into my clinic as a muscle relaxant. Related defects when taken during pregnancy include cleft palate, club-foot, neural tube defects, growth retardation, and subnormal intelligence quotient.[60] Research conducted in 2007 found that maternal use of carbamazepine was linked to foetal arteriovenous malformations, cardiovascular teratogenicity, and anticonvulsant syndrome.[61]

- **Antacid or acid-lowering medications**
These are prescribed to relieve reflux and heartburn—conditions often experienced during pregnancy. There are several concerns associated with lowering stomach acid, which include impaired breakdown of protein in the stomach; impaired absorption of essential nutrients, including vitamin B12, iron, calcium, magnesium, and zinc; and impaired release of digestive enzymes and bile. Poor bile flow can lead to gall stones, which is explained more in section II. Low stomach acid levels not only impair

nutrient breakdown and absorption but also affect the pH balance (acid/alkaline balance) of the small intestine, which can lead to bacterial overgrowth. Long-term use of antacids can result in osteoporosis, developing *Helicobacter pylori* bacterial infection, malnutrition, and mental health conditions.[62] As your growing baby relies on the nutrients you consume in food, it's best not to impair the digestive process in any way. You'll find suggestions on relieving reflux and heartburn in section II.

- **Alcohol**
Clinical trials as far back as 1968 have clearly established the link between prenatal ethanol exposure and birth defects, termed foetal alcohol syndrome (FAS).[63] Despite the hundreds of clinical, epidemiological, and experimental studies undertaken over the years, alcohol consumption during gestation remains socially acceptable. Abnormalities associated with FAS fall into three major categories—growth retardation, mental retardation, and neurological abnormalities with craniofacial dysmorphism including microcephaly. Abnormalities associated with FAS also extend to organs of the cardiovascular system, liver, kidney, genitals, cutaneous membranes, musculature, skeletal tissue, and neural tube and have also been known to cause tumours.

Embryonic and foetal nutrient supplies are significantly impaired by drugs that inhibit circulation through the placenta. Delivery of oxygen to the foetus occurs via the umbilical blood flow, and hypoxia has been associated in increased foetal mortality, malformations, and growth retardation. Impaired blood flow also increases free radical damage to the delicate embryonic tissues by compromising cell membrane integrity. Therefore, any drugs inhibiting circulation through the placenta impact embryonic and foetal nutrient supplies. Impaired placental circulation would not only impact nutrient flow to the foetus but also delay clearance of waste products, leading to toxicity within the developing baby. Adequate nutrition has become the focus of increasing studies revealing that programming of future health begins long before birth.[64] Ethanol has been shown to interfere with digestion and absorption of nutrients, in particular zinc, folate, and pyridoxine; vitamins A and D; and magnesium, while tissue concentrations of iron and manganese are elevated with chronic alcohol intake. Ethanol has also been shown to interfere with essential fatty acid metabolism and prostaglandin synthesis in the embryo.

- **Vitamin A**
Vitamin A reflects a group of retinoids, which are best consumed as compounds (in foods) rather than isolates (synthetic supplements). These retinoids are required for normal growth, vision, sperm formation, red blood cells, immunity, and mucous membranes as found in the respiratory and digestive tracts.[65] However, excessively high levels of vitamin A have been shown to have teratogenic actions when total consumption exceeds 10,000 IU per day of preformed retinol, whereas vitamin A derived from beta-carotene is not associated with birth defects. Teratogenic action is dependent on the embryonic or foetal developmental stage, quality of retinoid compound consumed, and dosage taken. Higher doses, increasing frequency, and severity of defects are attributed to embryo death. Overexposure during embryonic development has been linked to craniofacial and overt central nervous system defects.[66]

Just as excess vitamin A may be teratogenic, insufficient levels of this vitamin impact negatively on the development of foetal mucosa that originated from endodermal tissue. Vitamin A deficiency during pregnancy increases the baby's susceptibility to infections.[67] It also increases the risk of the mother developing eclampsia and premature rupture of membranes.[68] The effect of vitamin A on mucosal membranes may be a relevant consideration in light of Australia's high incidence of respiratory ailments, in particular asthma.

Retinol forms of vitamin A are found in animal foods like cod liver oil, salmon, egg yolks, butter, and liver, while beta-carotene is found in yellow, orange, and some green leafy vegetables but mainly sweet potatoes, pumpkin, carrots, capsicum, and beetroot. By cooking vegetables, you can lose up to 35 per cent of this important nutrient.

Vitamin A supports healthy mucous membranes—think lungs and digestive system—but it also supports a healthy immune system, maintains the myelin sheath that surrounds nerve cells, helps prevent birth defects, is involved in vision, and increases iron utilisation. Our body cannot produce any form of this vitamin, which makes it an essential nutrient we must get from our diet. Vitamin A's reputation as dangerous during pregnancy has come about due to over-supplementation, rather than dietary excesses. It also works in tandem with vitamin D, which is why foods containing one often also contain the other.

A better understanding of the dangers of various substances including alcohol, medications, and some nutrients may assist in reducing drug-related birth defects. Substances ingested by a woman are of particular relevance during the first weeks of gestation. Often during these fateful first weeks, the woman is oblivious to being pregnant. They say knowledge is power, and when it comes to what you are exposing yourself to, this definitely fits.

It should also be noted that natural medicine offers viable support for many of the symptoms mentioned above. Rather than reaching for a quick-fix painkiller or decongestant, consider visiting your local naturopath. Not only does nature offer many safe options, but looking deeper at what is causing your symptoms may actually lead to total resolution of the problem you are seeking to treat with medications.

How to reduce your exposure to gender-bender chemicals

Awareness is the first step to reducing your exposure to toxic substances. By following a few easy steps, you can make great inroads to living a more toxin-free life. Although this is important for everyone, pregnant women and women who may become pregnant, as well as men seeking to father a healthy baby, should pay particular attention to reducing their exposure as much as possible. Change is rarely easy, and changing lifelong habits can be both daunting and challenging. Begin with small changes you can manage easily. Acknowledge the successes you have along the way. And don't become discouraged if you revert to old habits. Refocus and start again. Keep your goal in mind—having a healthy baby.

1. As much as possible, choose organic fruit and vegetables, as well as organic / free-range meats, poultry, and eggs to reduce exposure to pesticides, fertilisers, antibiotics, and growth promotants used in agriculture and animal husbandry.
2. Rather than eating farmed fish, which are often heavily contaminated with EDCs, PCBs, antibiotics, and mercury, supplement with a high-quality purified fish or seaweed oils, or eat fish that is wild-caught. Smaller fish varieties contain less mercury.
3. Eat mostly whole, fresh foods, steering clear of processed, pre-packaged foods of all kinds. This way you automatically avoid artificial additives, including dangerous artificial sweeteners, food colouring, and MSG.
4. Store your food and beverages in glass rather than plastic and avoid using plastic wrap—or ensure it does not touch your food.
5. Have your tap water tested. If contaminants are found, install an appropriate water filter or a whole-of-house filter to ensure clean water from all taps (even those in your shower or bath—this is particularly important for your baby).
6. Avoid using artificial air fresheners, dryer sheets, fabric softeners, or other synthetic fragrances, replacing these with quality essential oils.
7. Replace your Teflon pots and pans with quality stainless steel or stoneware.
8. When renovating your home, look for "green", toxin-free alternatives in lieu of regular paint and vinyl floor coverings.

***

Healthy habits are learned in the same way as unhealthy ones—
through practice.
—Wayne W. Dyer

How toxic is your life: A quick personal self-assessment

Almost half of the women (45 per cent) in a study conducted at Boise University, Idaho, considered there was no risk in using cosmetics during pregnancy, although "it is now recognized that these products contain numerous potentially harmful chemical substances including plasticizers, bisphenol A, parabens, synthetic dyes, benzophenones, antimicrobials, dioxane, formaldehyde and heavy metals."[69] If you regularly use any of the following personal care care items or household products, chances are your body is challenged by a build-up of toxins. Tick the items you use on a regular basis—you may be surprised at just how many chemicals you are exposing yourself to daily.

Personal care

- ☐ Shampoo
- ☐ Conditioner
- ☐ Soap
- ☐ Body wash
- ☐ Bubble bath
- ☐ Make-up remover
- ☐ Hair-spray
- ☐ Hair gel / mousse
- ☐ Hair colour / dyes / perms
- ☐ Acne creams
- ☐ Antibacterial soaps
- ☐ Hand cream / body lotions / moisturiser
- ☐ Sunscreen
- ☐ Shaving cream
- ☐ Aftershave lotion
- ☐ Antiperspirant / deodorant
- ☐ Nail polish
- ☐ Nail polish remover
- ☐ Gel nails
- ☐ Tattoos
- ☐ Make-up
- ☐ Lipstick / lip gloss
- ☐ Perfume
- ☐ Baby wipes / Wet Ones

Household items

- ☐ Dishwasher and dishwashing detergent
- ☐ Dishwasher final rinse aid
- ☐ Chlorine-containing cleaners, bleach
- ☐ Air fresheners
- ☐ Weed-killing sprays, especially glyphosate
- ☐ Spray cleaners
- ☐ Laundry powder
- ☐ Fabric softener
- ☐ Pesticide sprays

You may argue that surely our governments would not permit toxic substances to be sold. The truth is the control of toxic substances does not lie with an independent body. While manufacturers are required to test many of the chemicals used in their products, these are tested individually and at low concentrations. However, if you use any of the above items more often than once in your lifetime, chances are toxins have built up in your body. Further, it is the combination of chemicals together and long-term use that exacerbates the toxicity problem we are experiencing today.

Is your job toxic?

Where we work often also poses considerable challenges for our body. Here are a few professions that increase your exposure to toxic chemicals:

- Hairdressers
- Nail technicians
- Beauticians
- Metal trades workers
- Maritime trades workers
- Timber trades workers
- Builders
- Plasterers
- Painters
- Motor vehicle mechanics
- Spray painters
- Farmers
- Greens keepers – golf courses, bowling greens

Many of the above positions involve repeated exposure to toxic substances. There are, of course, lots of others. But some of the above aren't commonly thought of as being toxic workplaces. Always wear protective clothing and remember that exposed skin can absorb chemicals, so cover up.

How do you avoid toxins?

Clean up your bathroom and kitchen. These two rooms harbour the most toxic substances used in homes.

- Use only natural, chemical-free body care products. Read the labels and familiarise yourself with the chemicals used.

- Avoid using any commercial baby care products—keep your baby free of toxins as much as possible to avoid your little one developing allergies and other chronic health conditions. Organic coconut oil is wonderful on baby's delicate skin.
- Use natural, earth-friendly cleaning products in your home. There is no need to have a different product for different areas of your home. There is no need to use harsh cleaners. Vinegar, baking soda, borax, washing soda, and essential oils provide natural protection from bacteria and viruses. Check online for instructions on how to easily make your own natural cleaning products or select from the many new brands that provide safe cleaning.
- Open windows and doors—good airflow will help rid your home of odours, as well as keep the mould/mildew at bay.
- Invest in a dehumidifier and/or air purifier.
- If you have a garden, refer to organic and natural gardening websites for great tips on how to avoid toxic sprays. Learn about companion planting to reduce pests.

Remember, every chemical you remove from your life will benefit you and your family.

How can I test if I'm toxic?

There are various functional medicine tests available to assess your body's level of toxicity. Perhaps the easiest, fastest, and least costly is the hair tissue mineral analysis (HTMA), where a small sample of clean hair is assessed for mineral content and presence of heavy metals. Hair is an effective medium, as our body deposits both minerals and heavy metals into tissue, of which hair is the most easily accessible.

People often ask me if blood can reveal whether their body has heavy metals or to check nutrient status. Blood is a poor indicator of both nutrient and toxin levels. Blood is a transport medium, which carries nutrients, oxygen, and other substances to our cells. When we want to know how our body is doing, we really need to assess the level of nutrients (or toxins) located in our cells, tissues, and organs. As it's not easy (nor pain-free) to take a tissue sample from inside the body, we use hair.

Nutrients like calcium and magnesium are stored in tissues—calcium is predominantly stored in bones and teeth, while magnesium is mostly stored in the muscles. Both these and other minerals are essential for many functions carried out daily. So, when availability drops, our body starts to draw on tissue stores. Signs of insufficient minerals include osteoporosis—a lack of calcium in bones—or muscle cramping due to low magnesium levels. Likewise, heavy metals and other toxins tend to be stored in tissue. Lead has an affinity for bones, while mercury accumulates in the kidneys, eyes, brain, thyroid gland, and liver. Other heavy metals cause problems by displacing or blocking essential nutrients, preventing them from being used for biochemical processes throughout the body.

Another useful method to measure toxins is to assess what your body is excreting. Urine is an excellent medium to test both nutritional levels and toxicity. When assessing urine, the laboratories identify how your body is carrying out the many biochemical processes that occur daily. Tests available include organic acids test (OAT), which offers a comprehensive metabolic snapshot of a patient's overall health with over seventy markers. Various other tests for toxic substances, including mould, over 170 toxic chemicals, and glyphosate are available.

While we're on the topic of testing, functional medicine assessment of hormones and how your body processes these can also be useful, especially if you are experiencing fertility or conception problems. All these tests and recommended laboratories are listed in Appendix 3.

Signs and symptoms of toxicity

Diverse symptoms may indicate toxicity, including headaches/migraines, obesity/weight gain, inability to lose weight, nausea, poor concentration/memory, fatigue/lethargy, skin problems, fluid retention, muscle stiffness or pain, low mood, puffiness under the eyes, digestive discomfort, excessive perspiration, allergies, infertility, and pain. You may even be symptom-free until such time as you "suddenly" develop a debilitating illness.

It's always best to avoid toxins, but if this is not possible, then give your body all the support it needs to clear them from your system. Don't be tempted to purchase an off-the-shelf detox product—these can do more harm than good.

How do I clean out my body?

If you find you have accumulated heavy metals or other chemicals, don't fret. There are ways to help your body clear these. I must stress, though, that doing a three-day detox with the aid of an over-the-counter product is not recommended. Nor are extreme water or juice fasts. Any toxins that have accumulated in your body have most likely done so over a period of time, mostly many years. They cannot be pulled out of cells and tissues quickly. For example, lead displaces calcium in bones, so removing lead quickly would leave your bones severely depleted of calcium.

Before undertaking any form of detoxification, you must ensure that all elimination pathways (bowels, kidneys, lymphatics, lungs, and skin) are functioning optimally. You don't want to go stirring up a whole lot of chemicals, causing a toxic soup to circulate in your body. Therefore, this is an area where I really stress the importance of consulting a qualified natural health practitioner or naturopath. There are no shortcuts, and a lot of damage can be caused if you try and do it yourself, although there are a few dietary changes you can make to help things along the way.

Often when I've discussed the need to detox with couples seeking to conceive, some were reluctant to put in the effort or the time. We all have things that are stored. And most toxins love fatty tissue—with the exception of lead, which gets stored in bones. Fatty tissue includes the ovaries, and follicle maturation takes about twelve months, so you begin to comprehend the need to thoroughly detox well before seeking to conceive. Chelation can take anywhere from six months to two years, depending on the toxin and duration of the exposure. But taking the time to clear heavy metals out of your body is well worth the effort and time invested, considering that exposure correlates with children being born with a disability. It is important to reassess toxicity every three months until clear for conception. Ultimately, parents must decide but need to understand the possible consequences for their children.

The liver is our major detoxification organ, filtering all the blood that passes through our body. If the liver is congested or sluggish, toxins will build up in the body, affecting the lymphatic and immune systems. To assist your lymphatic system, reduce foods known to increase congestion like dairy, refined carbohydrates, and sugar. The lymphatic system, unlike your blood, does not have a heart to pump it around the body—it relies on muscle action. So, keep active to help clear lymphatic congestion. Reduce liver irritants including alcohol and caffeine (coffee, tea, caffeinated soft drinks, and energy drinks). Try replacing coffee with dandelion tea—it looks and tastes very similar to coffee while supporting liver function. Eating your greens is highly beneficial and veggies including broccoli, Brussels sprouts, onions, and legumes, as well as eggs help provide the sulfur needed to help clear toxins. The fibre in vegetables can also assist in binding toxins in the digestive tract. Also, ensure you're drinking enough purified water every day to help flush out toxins.

While clearing out any stored toxins, it is essential that you avoid re-contamination. Refer back to the section on how you can reduce exposure to toxins, review your personal care products and household cleaners, be sure to use protective work wear, and incorporate organic foods in your diet.

Now that you have a really good understanding of environmental toxins, let's move onto another important topic—diet. Not all toxins can be avoided. However, ensuring sufficient levels of essential nutrients are present to offset the damaging effects may help protect the foetus and potentially reduce the risk of adverse foetal programming. These nutrients include vitamins and minerals.

***

- ❖ Each year, 4.5 billion litres of pesticides are sprayed on crops in Britain alone.
- ❖ Review your home and workplace for chemicals and remove those you can.
- ❖ Test for toxins and invest the time to clean up your body before conception.

5

Diet

> Let food be thy medicine and medicine be thy food
> —Hippocrates

What you eat is possibly the most important factor influencing health. And yet, it's frequently the most underestimated.

The word "diet" carries with it negative connotations, involving a period of time when certain foods are avoided, mostly to lose weight. However, "diet" from a nutritional perspective relates to the foods you consume daily on a regular basis. The choices you make about foods you consume should focus on foods being beneficial for your health and well-being, as well as the health of your future baby. In this book, when I refer to diet, it is definitely from a nutritional perspective.

So, why is it so difficult to eat our veg? Eating has become associated with the perception that it is a chore—a direct result of marketing and media advertising fast solutions. Takeaway has snuck into the lives of families to become a regular feature, rather than an occasional treat. The price for convenience and speed has cost us dearly, which is reflected in rising rates of obesity, illness, and infertility.

Changing the way and what we eat is a challenge just like any other long-term habit—let's face it, most of us have been eating the "modern" way since birth. By explaining a little more about the foods our body needs and why, I'm hoping to encourage you to take the first steps towards making more nutritious choices. After all, every mouthful you take is meant to nourish and nurture every single cell in your body and your future baby's body—do it for them.

Let's begin with the foods we eat and beverages we drink and what will support your baby's health, as well as what will not.

What's in the food we eat?

Foods we consume fall into one of two categories—macro and micronutrients. The macronutrients are protein, carbohydrates, and fats, while micronutrients include vitamins and minerals.

Protein

Protein is made up of twenty amino acids, and while all are important, nine are termed "essential"—meaning we need to consume these as part of our daily diet because our body cannot make them. The essential amino acids are building blocks for other amino acids and all our body tissues—which include bones, muscles, hair, skin, tendons, ligaments, blood, immune cells, hormones, neurotransmitters, all our organs, and our DNA structure. Amino acids also form methyl groups—more of which will be explained later under methylation.

The best-known sources of protein are animal products—meat, poultry, fish, eggs, and dairy. While plant foods also contain protein, these are generally at far lower quantities and often do not provide the full complement of all the essential amino acids. Plant foods providing a complete protein (that is, all nine essential amino acids) include quinoa, soy (remember, any soy product must be certified organic and non-GMO and, preferably, fermented as in tofu or tempeh), while beans, pulses, and nuts provide only some of the essential nine. It is for this reason that anyone seeking to follow a vegan diet should inform themselves on how best to combine foods to ensure they are consuming complete proteins. However, by combining two key plant categories you will get the complete protein—for example, 2 parts grain, nut, or seed + 1 part legume = complete protein. A guide to vegetarian and vegan eating is in Appendix 1.

During pregnancy the mother's protein requirement increases by about one-third or optimally between 18 per cent to 20 per cent of her total calorie intake.[70] To calculate your body's protein needs, use this easy calculation:

Your ideal body weight _____ kg x 0.8 = _____ grams of protein daily

If you prefer a vegetarian or vegan diet, the calculation is similar:

Your ideal body weight ____kg x 1.0 (vegetarian) or 1.2 (vegan) = ____ grams of protein required daily

During pregnancy, you may need to increase this amount by up to 30 per cent to meet the growing baby's needs.

Example. If you weigh 75 kg, then 75 x .08 = 60 grams of protein needed daily. If you are pregnant, you increase this by 25 per cent, so your protein need is now 75 grams of protein daily. Appendix 1 provides easy reference tables listing the protein content of foods to help you work out just how much protein is contained in the foods you eat.

Carbohydrates

The carbohydrates (carbs) that are most beneficial are those classified as "complex", which basically boils down to "whole" foods as opposed to "processed" foods. All plant foods provide carbs, which are essential for nutrients, fibre, and energy production. Plant foods include vegetables, fruit, whole grains, nuts, and seeds. Consider this—if you can look at a food and recognise what it is, it's a better option. A slice of an apple is recognisable as being part of an apple; the same can't be said about a fruit gummy.

The processing of grains has led to a reduction in fibre as well as nutritional content because the outer parts of the grains are removed—even wholemeal bread contains very little of the original grain. It is from whole carbs that we receive most of our vitamins and minerals, and whole grains provide essential nutrients for a healthy microbiome (more about the essential role these bugs play in our health and well-being later). When choosing plant foods, please consider sourcing organic, unsprayed, and definitely non-GMO produce to avoid all the toxic chemicals used in commercial agriculture.

Processed carbs, on the other hand, are low in nutritional value but high in sugars. And while these foods may give you a rush of energy, it is short-lived, leaving you needing more very soon. It is this cycle of highs and lows of sugar intake that lead to insulin resistance and can even culminate in type 2 diabetes. Carbs that contain high fibre along with natural sugars provide slower release and, therefore, sustained energy. Another term to know here is the "glycaemic index," which classifies foods into fast and slow sugar releasers. Fibre is a great way to slow a sugar "high." For example, having one or two organic dates with a handful of walnuts provides a sweet and nutritious snack while avoiding a peak in blood sugar levels.

Fibre, contained in plant foods, can support healthy cholesterol levels and reduce incidence of gall bladder disease and colon cancer. It assists in bowel transit time and may help prevent constipation (ensure you are consuming sufficient water) and support clearance of toxins from the bowel.

A recommended portion of your total calorie intake of complex carbs is 50 per cent or approximately 30 grams.

Fats

Fats have been demonised for several decades when the low-fat diet was touted as the answer to all our health problems. Then we were told to eat "good" fats. So, which are the "good" and which are the "bad" fats? Fats fall into various categories—saturated, hydrogenated, or trans-fats; polyunsaturated or mono-unsaturated fats; and essential fatty acids.

Fats are a source of long-term energy, especially for exercise that lasts longer than twenty minutes. In addition to providing energy, healthy fats play a vital role in hormone production and maintaining the integrity of cell membranes, especially nerve tissue. Only a small portion of your fat intake should be in the form of saturated fats from butter, dairy, and fatty meats. However, we do need that *small* amount, as saturated fats help our bodies clear out some heavy metals.

Saturated fats are mostly contained in animal products like meat, poultry, and dairy but are also found in coconut and palm oil. Some sources of unhealthy saturated fats you may not expect include cheese, ice cream and coffee creamer. Limit use of coconut oil to cooking, as it is stable at higher temperatures.

Unsaturated fats are those mainly derived from plants like nuts and seeds. But beware of hydrogenation, which creates trans-fats. This is the process by which a plant oil—seed or nut oils—are hydrogenated to become solid or spreadable. This is where the original concept for margarine came into being, but the process was flawed.

We now know hydrogenation causes fats to become sticky, increasing risk of heart disease, stroke, and diabetes—exactly the conditions that were previously blamed on butter and the reason margarine became so popular. Interestingly, the American FDA has declared that, after January 1, 2020, no food manufacturers are allowed to add partially hydrogenated oils to their foods.[71] However, keep checking ingredient labels for trans-fats, as this ruling may not apply in other countries.

Unsaturated fats are found in cooking oils, seeds, nuts, fish, and some vegetables. The two main types are mono and polyunsaturated oils. The monounsaturated oils suitable for low-temperature cooking include olive oil, peanut oil, and avocado oil. But oils are best added to food just before serving to preserve their nutritional value. The polyunsaturated fats include the omega-3, omega-6, and omega-9 oils.

Essential Fatty Acids

As with our essential amino acids, there are also essential fatty acids, which must be obtained from diet. Essential fatty acids (EFAs) include the omega-3 and omega-6 oils.[72] Omega-9 oils can be synthesised in the body and are not true "essential" fats. Omega-3 oils are contained in cold water fish, seaweed, flaxseeds/linseeds, pumpkin seeds, and black currant seeds. Sources of omega-6 oils include olive, sunflower, corn, and soybean oils; and sources of omega-9 oils include avocado, almond, peanut, and walnut oils. Given the amount of genetic modification, I recommend avoiding soy, corn, sunflower, and canola oils (as well as any products that contain any of these oils).

The essential components of omega-3 oils are

- eicosapentaenoic acid (EPA), beneficial for heart health and good circulation, supporting immune function, improving joint flexibility, healthy skin and hair, and cell membrane structure; and
- docosahexaenoic acid (DHA), beneficial for brain function, nervous system, pregnancy and foetal development, protecting the aging mind, improving behaviour, focus and learning in children, healthy eyes, and reducing harmful effects of stress.

It is these EFAs that help maintain healthy cell membranes while also promoting the body's natural anti-inflammatory response, a function that can relieve many chronic conditions, which are all too often inhibited by poor nutrition.

Studies associate higher intakes of EFAs during pregnancy with improved foetal growth and development during gestation.[73] DHA in particular plays a key role during foetal and infantile brain development acting on multiple levels, including healthy membrane growth, gene expression, protection against oxidative stress, and conduction of nerve impulses. DHA also supports the development of brain structure, contributing 30 per cent to 40 per cent of the total fatty acids within the grey matter of the cerebral cortex.[74] Additionally, DHA is involved in processes that support neuronal health, including regulation, protection, and repair.[75] Clean and pure fish oil providing 600 mg of DHA per day taken throughout gestation to birth improved infant growth and development, resulting in improved birth outcomes, although I recommend a combination of both EPA and DHA. Fish oil was also shown to improve foetal cardiac autonomic control, support eye health, and support newborn neuro-behaviour.

Fish oils also help the pregnant mum—you may think that baby brain is just an excuse for forgetfulness or being distracted. Well, let me impress on you that baby brain is very real. Just as EFAs support foetal brain development, they also help keep mum's brain functioning. Remember also that, as the foetus grows, it needs nutrients, and sometimes this can leave mum deficient—just another reason to maintain a healthy diet and take supplements if needed.

As with any supplement, quality is paramount, and this is particularly important when it comes to fish oils. You'll find recommended brands at the end of the book. For those who prefer a vegan source of omega-3 EFAs, I must explain that plant sources convert poorly into EPA and DHA. For example, only 1 per cent of linseed oil converts to DHA. At the time of writing, the only reputable vegan source is one made from algae. Furthermore, it is best that men avoid taking high doses of flaxseed oil as a source of EFA while its testosterone-lowering effects are better researched. A most important note: *Always keep your EFA oils refrigerated.*

Our intake of omega-3 and omega-6 oils should be roughly equal, but typical western diets are slanted toward significantly higher omega-6 consumption, which can lead to inflammatory conditions. Try using black sesame seed oil on salads instead of olive oil for a balance of omega-3, 6, and 9 oils.

Vitamins and minerals

Vitamins are either water or fat soluble—water-soluble vitamins need to be replenished daily, while the fat-soluble ones can be stored in the body. The fat-soluble vitamins include vitamins A, E, and D, although vitamin D is actually a hormone and not technically a true vitamin. Vitamin C is water soluble, as are the B complex group of vitamins, all of which are found in fruit and vegetables and some animal products. I have included a comprehensive table providing sources of each nutrient in Appendix 2 and more information on nutrients will be discussed in the chapter 12, "Nutrition for Mother and Baby."

Some of the better-known minerals include calcium, magnesium, iron, and zinc. Other minerals you may not be so familiar with include potassium, sodium, silicon, sulfur, manganese, selenium, copper, chromium, chloride, iodine, phosphorous, molybdenum, and boron. Each and every mineral is essential to your health in ensuring your body can function properly.

***

> "You can trace every sickness, every disease and every ailment to a mineral deficiency."
> —Linus Pauling, Nobel Prize-winner for chemistry in 1954, summing up the importance of minerals

6

The B Vitamins

You can never learn less, you can only learn more.
—R. Buckminster Fuller

I'd like to dedicate more space to this very special group of vitamins, as they are involved in many essential functions throughout the body. This group of vitamins includes seven varieties:

- B1, thiamine (thiamine pyrophosphate);
- B2, riboflavin (flavin adenine dinucleotide or FAD);
- B3, niacin (niacinamide or nicotinamide riboside);
- B5, pantothenic acid (calcium pantothenate);
- B6, pyridoxine (pyridoxal-5-phosphate or P-5-P);
- B9, folate (levomefolic acid, calcium folinate); and
- B12, cobalamin (hydroxo/methyl/adenosyl-cobalamin).

The descriptions in parentheses are the active form of each vitamin. The B vitamins are readily available from whole foods—including plant and animal products—and are used widely throughout the body for energy production, cardiovascular and nerve health. To list and explain all the functions could fill a book on its own. Suffice it to say, they are very important and, unfortunately, often insufficient in modern diets. B vitamins are depleted when taking the oral contraceptive pill and when under stress (including from electromagnetic frequencies). When supplementing, you should take the entire group in a B complex, rather than only taking one or two on their own.

Unfortunately, women are often prescribed folate (in its inactive form) on its own, rather than as part of a B complex. Another factor unbalancing the relationships between all our B vitamins is the fortification of highly processed foods with synthetic folate and thiamine.

Along with some amino acids, choline, and some other nutrients, the B vitamins are intricately involved in methylation.

Methylation

Methylation is a vital metabolic process that happens in every cell and every organ in your body, taking place a million times a second. Life would simply not exist without it. Think of billions of little on/off switches inside your body that control everything from your stress response and how your body makes energy from food to your brain chemistry and detoxification. That's methylation. It is the process by which the body makes enzymes that either support tissue generation (making or repairing tissue) or support detoxification. Methylation is a complex process, and if parts of what you are about to read seem like a foreign language, it is. Don't get hung up on all the weird terms and long words. Rather, try and understand the overall concept and appreciate how fundamental it is to your and your baby's health.

Methylation is a biochemical reaction that involves the transfer of a methyl group onto amino acids, proteins, enzymes, and DNA. Think of methyl groups as information messengers. The addition of a methyl group, which is made up of specific nutrients including choline, methionine, B6, B9, and B12, onto an amino acid facilitates a host of biochemical reactions, including

- more than 400 enzymatic and cellular reactions;
- DNA synthesis and repair;
- cell replication and repair (growth and healing);
- neurotransmitter synthesis and metabolism (mental health);
- energy production and metabolism;
- hormone regulation and fertility, including sperm DNA and sperm function;
- detoxification;
- epigenetics (gene expression and regulation); and
- telomere integrity (associated with the ageing process).

What else can influence methylation?

Because methylation takes place in every cell of your body, if it's not working properly, your health will be negatively impacted. When a wrong "switch" is flicked, causing changes, these can be minor to quite severe. But the outcome is that a particular function just won't happen the way it should.

SNPs (single nucleotide polymorphisms) are the most common type of genetic variation among people. Each SNP (pronounced /snip/) represents a modification in a single DNA building block, called a nucleotide. Some of the more common ones include MTHFR (involving folate), COMT (brain function), MAO (neurotransmitters), PEMT (choline), as well as SNPs affecting detoxification and antioxidants. The best way to assess any SNPs you and your partner may have is with a quality DNA test that identifies and reports on your SNPs rather than just providing fancy images and possible health complications. Knowing how to support your body and circumvent any SNPs you may have can greatly influence the outcome of having a healthy baby—well worth the investment in a good DNA test.

Pregnancy is a critical time, during which DNA methylation can shape neonatal health outcomes by regulating healthy gestational development and genetic expression.[76] Inadequate methylation is a contributing factor in many disease states; however, nutrients that act as methyl donors can promote healthy methylation.[77] Adequate consumption of choline provides 60 per cent of the body's methyl groups[78] by serving as a precursor for S-adenosylmethionine (SAMe) production—the universal methyl donor in the body. Genetic polymorphisms related to impaired methylation have been linked to the accumulation of homocysteine, which is associated with adverse outcomes in pregnancy, including neural tube defects (NTDs), poor foetal brain development, preeclampsia, and miscarriage.[79] Ensuring an adequate supply of methylating nutrients, including choline and vitamins B6, B9, and B12 before and throughout pregnancy may help methylation and safeguard better health outcomes. Methylation throughout pregnancy fluctuates, but demands are highest during the developmental phases occurring between weeks fifteen to seventeen. If there are insufficient nutrients to support methylation, the mother may experience symptoms of exhaustion and depression.

Nutritional sources of choline include beans, beef and chicken liver (definitely only organic), egg yolks (organic), lentils, lecithin, split peas, organic/non-GMO soybeans, spinach, some whole grains, and yeast. For more information on sources of nutrients, refer to Appendix 2.

What is MTHFR?

Methylenetetrahydrofolate reductase is an enzyme that adds a methyl group to folic acid to make it usable by the body. You could think of this enzyme as activating your credit card—unless activated, you can't use it. The same applies to folic acid. The MTHFR gene is the recipe needed to make this enzyme, which is required for converting folic acid into its active form 5MTHF (5-methyltetrahydrofolate). This enzyme is also important for converting homocysteine into methionine—an essential sulfur amino acid critical for efficient detoxification. The SNP involved here is CBS. And to give you a little insight and understanding into why SNPs have such an impact on body functioning, let's have a quick look at what happens if this one enzyme is not working properly.

CBS is the first enzyme in the transsulfuration pathway and directs homocysteine away from methionine synthesis. Low methionine in turn can down-regulate CBS activity, which then impacts glutathione production. CBS activity produces hydrogen sulfide, which can protect the brain from hypoxia (low oxygen). CBS is expressed in the liver, brain, heart, lungs, kidneys, and pancreas in adults. In the foetus, it is expressed in the brain, liver, and kidneys. CBS is just one enzyme. But its effects on many different pathways of the body are significant. I hope this example helps you understand the complexities but, more importantly, the interactions between all functions that take place inside your body every second.

Back to folate—activated folate (5MTHF) goes on to give its methyl group to other nutrients and substances. This donation is known as methylation. Know that 5MTHF is required for the creation of every cell in your body—and every cell in your baby's body—and is also used to

- create neurotransmitters (serotonin, epinephrine, norepinephrine, and dopamine);
- create immune cells;
- process hormones (including oestrogen); and
- produce energy and detoxify chemicals.

Those with a defective MTHFR gene have an impaired ability to produce the MTHFR enzyme (estimates range from 20 per cent to 70 per cent). This can make it more difficult to break down and eliminate substances like heavy metals. Individuals with the MTHFR gene mutation have difficulties processing B9 in the synthetic form (commonly present in inferior supplements and added to processed foods). This type of B9 may even cause a build-up in the body leading to toxicity, which can raise homocysteine levels.

Elevated homocysteine is associated with a higher risk of heart disease, inflammation, birth defects, difficult pregnancies, and potentially an impaired ability to detoxify. This also affects the conversion to glutathione, which the body needs to remove waste, and which is our second-most potent antioxidant. Many factors can contribute to the expression of the MTHFR mutation, including our environment, foods, chemical exposure, and stress.

How do we get this mutation?

Variations in the specific genes can be passed on from each parent. If both parents pass on a healthy gene, the baby won't inherit a mutation. If one parent passes on a healthy gene but the other passes on a mutated gene (heterozygous), several variations can occur. If both parents pass on a mutated form (homozygous), there are many more scenarios that can result. But recall how the woman's egg, if healthy and sound, can repair any sperm defects to prevent the passing on of SNPs.

Gene variations can also be caused by environmental factors or epigenetics in the baby after birth and during its life. There are several other SNPs affecting folate, which are not as notorious as MTHFR but play equally important roles. These include MTHFD1 and SHMT1. In addition, MTR and MTRR involve B12, which along with B6 can affect methylation. So, when selecting a DNA assessment, ensure that the above SNPs are included.

I was asked whether it is possible for parents to change the SNPs they pass on to their children. What is passed on genetically is a code. If a child inherits a code, for example, G1958A on the MTHFD1 gene this will be the case forever. Understanding the impact of this function, however, enables parents to ensure the child's diet is adequate in folate and choline to prevent any adverse health outcomes in that child's future. What we can do is ensure that our and our children's DNA does not undergo any further unwanted alteration by ensuring good nutrition and avoiding toxins.

Food and its individual nutrients do more than just provide building blocks for our body's various structural and functional components. Food also communicates with our genes. Every mouthful of food sets off a complex conversation with the DNA in our cells, determining whether the protective or disease-promoting cellular "switches" are activated. This cellular communication by our foods is called nutrigenomics, a term coined in 2004 borne out of an understanding of how nutrients and other food-derived molecules impact cell function—and overall body health and well-being. Nutrigenomics can also be explained that food is medicine, just like Hippocrates said nearly 2,500 years ago.

***

- ❖ Methylation happens in every single cell of your body.
- ❖ Your child's DNA methylation patterns are established around day nine.
- ❖ Food communicates with your DNA.

7
Genes and Epigenetics

> Genetics load the gun and the environment pulls the trigger
> —Francis Collins

In other words, while your genes determine the colour of your eyes and other structural features, it is your behaviours, lifestyle, and environment that impact health outcomes. The term "environment" refers to both our external environments (what we are exposed to) and our internal environments (what's going on inside our bodies; think of this as how well your body is functioning and how effectively it can eliminate toxins). The field of science known as epigenetics—meaning above or over the gene—has enabled us to learn how important our diet and daily choices are for health outcomes. Furthermore, it empowers us to take active control of these factors, so we can literally help determine our health and genetic destiny, as well as that of our children.

Knowing that everything you consume affects how your mind and body function on a structural and functional level, as well as understanding how this influences your genes should help you make wiser choices when it comes to diet and lifestyle.

So, what is the best diet?

If I had to answer with just one word, it would be *clean*. People have many different preferences—from an omnivorous to variations of vegetarian, vegan, paleo, keto, or blood type diets. Whatever your personal choice of diet, everything you consume should be clean. By that, I mean grown organically without the use of pesticides, herbicides, antibiotics, and growth promotants; minimally processed; and free from GMO-ingredients, preservatives, and artificial additives.

Human beings evolved all over the planet, in different climatic and geographical zones. In some cultures, there was a balance between animal protein—meat, fish, eggs, and poultry—and plant foods, including vegetables, fruit, nuts, seeds, and grains. Other cultures, like the Inuit, consume predominantly fish, with very limited plant foods. Populations known to reach the highest age live in the "blue zones," which are located around the world.[80] But what they all have in common is the consumption of locally sourced fruit and vegetables and organically raised livestock, often eating between 70 and 90 per cent plant-based diets.

However, I must explain that "plant-based" does not mean manufactured meat imposters from plants, especially soy. Recent research has revealed that inflammatory biomarkers are higher in vegan "meat" products than in animal-based meats.[81] To clarify—eating clean represents eating foods grown and raised as nature intended, with a noted absence of chemicals, processing, and sugar.

As with the Mediterranean diet, there is a tendency for the blue zone cultures to come together and share mealtimes, illustrating that "how" we eat is as important as "what" we eat.

What you need to consider in addition to eating clean, is consuming a varied diet. It's all about the nutrients, which is of particular concern for people on any restrictive diet. For example, some nutrients are often deficient in vegan diets—especially vitamin B12, vitamin D, iron, and omega-3.[82] It is important to seek the advice and guidance of a qualified naturopath to avoid nutritional deficiencies if you need to be on a restricted diet. It is also essential that you read the ingredients on any product you purchase. You'd be surprised what has been added to that crumbed fish cutlet or ready-made lasagne or vegan "hamburger." The ingredients of many processed foods (which includes anything in a packet, can, jar, or bottle) include genetically modified wheat, soy, corn, canola oil, and more. Avoid these products unless the label specifically states that the product is free from GMO ingredients.

To help you understand some of those names and numbers on product ingredients lists, you might like to purchase the book *Chemical Maze* by Bill Stratham.[83] Or download the app so you have it with you when shopping. I often wonder what the person monitoring the supermarket security cameras thinks when they see me taking an item off the shelf, reading the ingredients, shaking my head in disgust, and replacing it. You, too, will be horrified at some of the ingredients in seemingly innocuous food products.

While chemicals are tested for toxicity to establish "safe" levels, they are rarely, if ever, tested in conjunction with others or over the longer term (the synergistic effect of several chemicals far outweighs the effect of the single components). If our bodies are constantly exposed, toxicity levels and detrimental effects accumulate and compound over time.

In addition to eating clean and sourcing fresh whole foods, how do you balance your nutritional needs?

As a general guide, your meals should consist of one-quarter protein, one-quarter grains or starches, and half vegetables.[84] This book does not provide the space for me to include meal plans, so I recommend you visit 40 Weeks, an online guide to nutrition during pregnancy (www.40weeks.com.au) for nutrient-dense recipes, as well as meal plans developed specifically to support the mum-to-be throughout pregnancy. There are also thousands of recipes easily accessible online. Just enter the key ingredients you would like to use, and *presto*, you'll have multiple recipes to choose from and adapt depending on your refrigerator or pantry contents. I've also included a few of my favourite recipe authors in Appendix 5.

Research in Germany found that a diet incorporating at least 600 grams of non-starchy vegetables and fruit daily was associated with the most health benefits.[85] Consuming 600 grams of vegetables and fruit a day may sound like a lot, but it actually isn't. Divide this over the course of three meals and snacks, varying the produce you have every day. Here's a fun challenge for you to see just how many different plant foods you consume over a week. Make a list of all the ingredients of the foods you eat. However, you can only list an ingredient/food once, regardless of how often you eat it. For example, if you have an apple every day, you can only list apple once. Remember this exercise is about variety. I've included a sample form and instructions in Appendix 1.

The modern foods

Our diets remained largely the same for thousands of years—consuming local produce. Depending on region, this included a variety of plant-based as well as animal foods. However, over the past hundred years, our diets have radically changed with the introduction of high-density industrialised agriculture, feed-lots for cattle, concrete stalls for pigs, and ponds for fish and seafood farming. This has been accompanied by widespread use of chemicals—artificial fertilisers, pesticides, herbicides, antibiotics, and growth promotants. Genetically modified corn has become a staple of livestock—animals that naturally feed on green pastures. Remember, everything your food has been exposed to enters your body—this includes all the chemicals and toxins.

Add to this the rise of highly processed "foods" from the mid-twentieth century, and you can begin to appreciate how our diet has been radically altered. Rather than consuming a varied diet of fresh/whole/seasonal foods, we have changed to eating highly processed, nutritionally deficient, highly modified toxic "food" imposters.

Commonly used additives in industrial and consumer foods include
- salt and MSG;
- sugars and intense sweeteners, including high-fructose corn syrup;
- gluten and transglutaminase, a texturising agent that mimics gluten;
- solvents including alcohol; and
- emulsifiers, including lecithin from genetically modified soy and sunflowers.

Many of these additives erode the lining of your digestive tract, increasing permeability, which leads to foreign substances entering the body activating autoimmune responses. Research shows that food additives are driving autoimmunity.[86]

Perhaps one of the most common additives used in a variety of foods and beverages is high-fructose corn syrup (HFCS). It is an inexpensive sweetener made from genetically modified corn and is used in soft drinks, juices, sweets (lollies and candy), breakfast cereals, baked goods, and snack foods. HFCS is linked to abdominal obesity, diabetes, cardiovascular disease, and non-alcoholic fatty liver disease (NAFLD), which has rapidly become the most common form of chronic liver disease in children and adolescents.

Another hidden additive that impacts greatly on mental health is MSG or monosodium glutamate. MSG is a flavour enhancer often added to restaurant foods, canned vegetables, soups, deli meats, frozen and other foods. It can cause symptoms including headache, sweating, numbness, flushing, rapid fluttering heartbeats, chest pain, and nausea. The glutamate component is also an excitatory neurotransmitter, which can exacerbate behavioural issues including ADD and ADHD. Excitotoxins are substances added to foods and beverages that literally stimulate neurons to death, causing brain damage of varying degrees. Excitotoxins can be found in ingredients such as MSG, aspartame, cysteine, hydrolysed protein, and aspartic acid.[87]

While both HFCS and MSG are required to be listed on product labels, they will go unnoticed if you don't diligently check the label on everything you purchase. Even if you've been using a particular brand for a while, it is wise to double-check because ingredients can change. These are just two of the hidden nasties in many foods we consume on a regular basis.

I recall a patient once commenting to me after I recommended eliminating processed tomato sauce and explaining my reasons. She said, "But if it weren't good for us, the government would not allow it to be sold in stores."

Unfortunately, her naivety is not an isolated example. Many people believe that what we are sold must be "approved" and be "good" for us. Nothing could be further from the truth. Professors David Raubenheimer and Stephen J. Simpson explain how ultra-processed foods no longer resemble anything we have eaten in the past. Fibre and protein have been removed or replaced, resulting in higher consumption to meet our nutrient needs. They write, "What do ice cream, chocolate, paint, shampoo, and crude oil all have in common? Answer: the science behind them." Interestingly, despite advances in modern medicine throughout the 1900s, the world disease levels have not declined. Obesity has taken over, correlating with the introduction of ultra-processed foods.

Animals should be raised outdoors on pastures that are spray-free, on soils that have not been eroded and over-fertilised. Vegetables and all plant foods should be grown organically without exposure to pesticides, herbicides, and chemical fertilisers. Always ask where your food comes from. While your local supermarket may not be able to provide this information other than country of origin, your local farmer or markets should know. It is well worth the effort to source locally grown produce. Some of our major cities have amazing markets, with smaller versions popping up in other urban areas. There is always the option of online ordering, growing your own, or starting a community garden.

Eating clean is especially important when it comes to seafood. In the name of sustainability, much is now grown in ponds. Consider that fish like barramundi, salmon, and tuna are hunters eating other fish; yet when farmed, they are often fed pellets of dubious content. Shellfish (prawns, crab, lobster, and bugs) and molluscs (mussels and oysters) are either bottom-feeders or reliant on tidal movement, but both take in toxins from their environment. For this reason, it is essential to know where your seafood comes from but also to only consume it very occasionally and consider avoiding it altogether during pregnancy.

What you consume is very important—for your own health and for the health of your microbiome. And it is also essential for the health of your child.

Supplements

In an ideal world, people everywhere would be able to obtain the nutrition they require from diet alone. So many factors make this unrealistic in our modern world. The quality of our soils is not what it used to be. Soil depleted of nutrients, trace minerals, and healthy soil microbes has a direct impact on plant, animal, and human health. In addition to lowered nutrient content of foods grown today, our needs have increased, driven by stress and constant exposure to toxins. Pregnancy also increases the body's need for nutrients. Always consult a qualified naturopath or natural health professional for guidance relating to supplements—quality is the key.

Some fundamental supplements that may be indicated during the preparation phase for both parents-to-be and throughout pregnancy/breastfeeding include B complex vitamins, fish oils, and a multimineral formulation or individual minerals, depending on need, such as zinc or iron. Unfortunately, due to guidelines of the TGA (the Australian Therapeutic Goods Administration), qualified practitioners, which includes naturopaths and nutritionists, are prohibited from recommending or naming TGA- approved therapeutic remedies outside of a clinical consultation. Sadly, unqualified people (including "influencers" and multilevel marketing organisations) are not governed by these censorship laws. So, my request to you is always to seek the advice of a qualified professional, as they are best equipped to assess your individual needs and recommend quality products.

You are not only feeding yourself

Given the theme of this book, you would be excused for thinking the section title refers to you also feeding your baby. However, in this instance, this is not my focus. Rather, I am referring to feeding your microbiome—all those tiny microbes that inhabit your digestive tract, without which we would not be able to extract the nutrients from the foods we eat.

***

- ❖ Take control of your health and genetic destiny.
- ❖ Eating 600 grams of non-starchy vegetables and fruit daily is associated with the most health benefits.
- ❖ If you're supplementing, then only high-grade quality is good enough.

8

Gut Health

> You are the foods you consume *and* the information that you digest.
> —Michael Corthell

Whether you say "gut," "tummy," "intestines," "bowel," or "digestive system," all these expressions refer to what is termed the gastrointestinal tract, or GIT. And it could be argued that it is the most important system in your body. Hippocrates knew what he was about when he said, "All disease begins in the gut."

How the gut works

Everything you consume passes through your gut. The GIT is where food is broken down—starting in the mouth with chewing food and salivary enzymes and then progressing into the stomach, where acid breaks down proteins and some carbs. Having good levels of stomach acid (hydrochloric acid) is essential for a healthy digestive system (this is why antacids cause huge problems if taken long term). The chyme (munched-up food from the stomach) enters the duodenum—the first section of your small intestine, where alkalising enzymes from the pancreas and bile from the gall bladder are added to the mix. It is in the small intestine where most of the nutrients are extracted and absorbed; however, a few nutrients and excess water are absorbed in the large intestine.

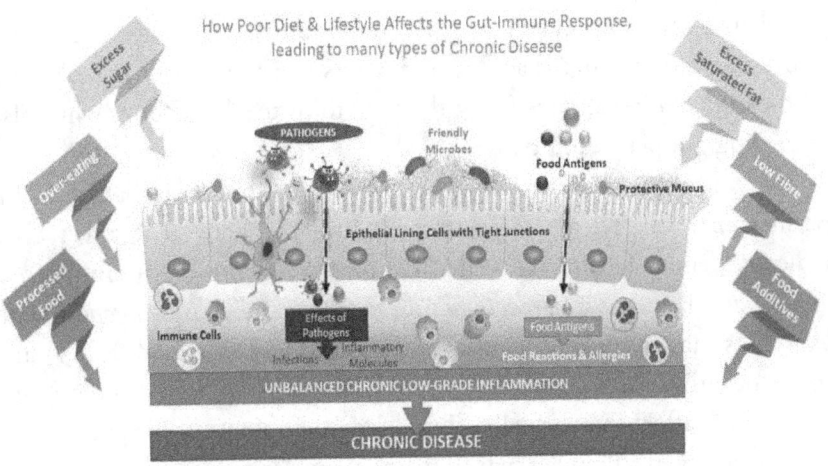

Table 3[88] shows how what we eat affects the integrity of the gut lining (epithelial cells), resulting in permeability or leaks admitting pathogens (bad bugs, bacteria, and parasites) and undigested food particles into the area behind the gut wall. These intruders create an immune response, leading to inflammation, food reactions, intolerances, and even allergies. Left unchecked, this can culminate in chronic disease, including autoimmune conditions.

In recent years, much research has been done into the microbiome—in particular those bacteria that reside in our gut and that play an integral role in a healthy, functioning digestive system. The effect of antibiotics on destroying important "good" bugs has become more widely known. Unfortunately, we do not only expose our microbiome to destructive antibiotics when prescribed by our doctor. The animal husbandry industry is the largest consumer of antibiotics. So, unless you have always consumed certified organic meats, chicken, eggs, dairy products, and fish, chances are your personal microbiome has suffered significantly.

Looking after your microbes is also important because they help maintain a healthy environment inside your digestive tract. If the "bad" bugs take over, you can become quite unwell, with symptoms ranging from constipation or diarrhoea to mental health issues. Gut permeability (often referred to as "leaky gut") can lead to food intolerances, immune imbalances, and even autoimmune conditions. So, it's definitely in your interest to keep your bugs healthy and well nourished, especially if you experience any food-related sensitivities—most of which are due to gut imbalance, rather than the actual food. Stress also affects your microbiome, with elevated adrenaline fuelling the growth of the "bad" bugs while also increasing gut permeability.

In addition to food intolerances and immune imbalance, gut permeability can release toxic bacteria into the body that affect both male and female fertility, as well as the foetus. Bacteria, including *E. coli*, *Chlamydia trachomatis*, *Ureaplasma urealyticum*, and *Neisseria gonorrhoeae*, as well as many viruses, including EBV, CMV, HSV, HPV, HHV, and more, negatively affect the health of the prostate gland, testes, and urethra, all of which affect sperm quality. Impaired microbiome of the gut, urinary tract, and semen all impact male fertility.[89] Any leakage of toxins, bacteria, or viruses into the pelvic cavity makes its way into the bloodstream, affecting the rest of the body and, potentially, the foetus.

Your microbiome is as individual as you are, and the myriad of bacteria, viruses, and fungi help you break down food, aid in synthesising nutrients, support your immune system, and perform many other important bodily functions. These tiny organisms are integral to overall health and can help prevent many chronic diseases. Just as they look after us, we need to look after them. The microbiome develops in the first few years of life, nurtured particularly during vaginal birth and breastfeeding but also through the foods a baby eats and the environment it is exposed to.

You may be familiar with terms such as probiotics and prebiotics. Probiotics attempt to replenish a few of the beneficial strains of microbes in the gut. They have value following an illness or after taking medication but should always be prescribed by a qualified practitioner, as not all probiotics are beneficial in all situations. A healthy gut has around a thousand different strains of microbes; taking up to fifteen is not going to rebalance your microbiome. Only a healthy gut and healthy diet can achieve this, and taking a probiotic supplement long term can actually result in damage to this intricately balanced microbial world inside you.

Prebiotics are foods that nourish your microbiome. Fibre contained in plant foods, especially vegetables but also healthy grains, is a source of food for your microbiome. The greater the variety and diversity of prebiotic rich foods, the healthier your microbiome will be. Generally, 30 to 50 grams of dietary fibre are recommended, and most of this will be provided when you eat 600 grams of non-starchy vegetables daily. Select a variety from the following to nurture and protect your healthy gut microbes—leeks, onions, garlic, spring onions, asparagus, globe artichoke, banana, lentils, chickpeas, nuts, apples, stone fruits, carrots, sweet potato (a note here—please choose organic and keep the skins on), oats, barley, flaxseed flakes, sesame seeds, rye, brown rice, organic non-GMO corn, unripe Lady Finger bananas, and cooked and cooled white potatoes with skins on. Cooking and cooling starchy foods like potatoes and rice changes the starch to a beneficial fibre. You'll find a list of common foods and fibre content in Appendix 2.

Eating small quantities of fermented foods like kimchi, sauerkraut, and kefir can also help to naturally populate your microbiome. There has been a significant rise in the popularity of kombucha drinks. I must impress on you that the cultures used do not have a shelf life. So, what remains is a very acidic drink, often high in sugar, which will contribute to unbalancing your body's pH while eroding tooth enamel.

I'd like to explain the concept of gut permeability as it directly relates to reproductive health. Intestinal permeability results when substances meant to be excreted "leak" into the pelvic cavity, affecting surrounding organs and even entering the bloodstream. Any toxins leaking out of the gut directly affect your reproductive organs—toxins are toxins, no matter where they come from. They impair how cells function. For the woman, this is particularly relevant if there are fertility issues but especially during pregnancy. The foetus receives nutrients via the placenta, which is directly linked to the maternal blood supply. So, if toxins from the gut have entered circulation, they will also enter the foetus.

As research continues into gut health, more information is coming to light. When gut microbes are unbalanced, they produce waste materials like phenols and aldehydes, both of which need to be cleared by the body in addition to all the other metabolic and environmental toxins. Both place added burden on the liver and cause other chemicals to build up—all in all, not a recipe for a healthy baby or an enjoyable pregnancy. Many common food additives have been linked to increasing gut permeability and autoimmunity. These include sugar, salt, intense sweeteners, alcohol, gluten, transglutaminase (undisclosed food texture excipient), emulsifiers, and nanoparticles.[90]

Once you conceive, gut-related issues should only be addressed under the supervision of a qualified naturopath. It is best to ensure your gut is healthy well prior to falling pregnant.

More about alcohol

As this book deals with having a healthy baby, it is advisable to limit your alcohol intake for at least six months prior to trying to conceive—and this goes for both parents. It takes six months to establish optimal oocyte and sperm health. By "limit," I mean one (regular) glass of quality, organic, additive-free wine up to twice a week with a meal. If you prefer beer, choose a quality brand that is free from additives and preservatives, and the same quantity applies—one glass or 375-millilitre bottle up to twice a week with food. Spirits, cocktails, and premixed drinks are best avoided. This is your investment in the health of your child, and you will benefit as well.

Remember to *stop all alcohol* once you decide you are ready to start "trying" to conceive. And definitely avoid alcohol entirely during pregnancy and while breastfeeding. Alcohol depletes minerals including calcium, magnesium, potassium, and zinc, as well as vitamins A, C, and B complex (especially B1 or thiamine). Furthermore, alcohol turns into acetaldehyde, which can damage DNA (yours and your baby's).[91] Boys born to mothers who consumed 4.5 drinks or more per week were found to have one-third lowered sperm count.[92] I really can't stress enough how everything you consume as parents-to-be affects your unborn baby.

***

- ❖ Healthy gut ↔ healthy microbiome = healthy body.
- ❖ Include naturally fermented foods in your diet like kimchi, sauerkraut, kefir.
- ❖ Consume fibre-rich whole fruits and vegetables daily.

9

The Importance of Water

> Pure water is the world's first and foremost medicine.
> —Slovakian proverb

Hydration! I can't stress this enough, as so many people are chronically dehydrated. Especially if you are looking to conceive, water is essential. Only a body that has sufficient water is able to function properly.[93] Pure, clean, filtered water is irreplaceable. Unfortunately, the water that comes out of our taps contains a lot of nasties—chlorine, fluoride, aluminium, and other heavy metals, as well as toxins from rain run-off, not to mention parasites and other microbes. Recycling water does not produce clean drinking water no matter what the authorities try and tell you. The amount of chemicals needed to treat sewage to produce "clean" water is phenomenal. In addition, hormones and medications cannot be removed from sewage, leading to a build-up in our water supplies. Bear in mind also that, if water is recycled and added to the main supply reservoirs, the environment and animal populations will be affected, as will you.

So, what about bottled water? Consider that most bottles are made of soft plastic, and you already have a source of oestrogen contamination. Commercial bottling plants must adhere to strict hygiene guidelines requiring sterilising the equipment with chlorine. Residues of chlorine and other chemicals may be found in bottled water. If you are unsure, have some brands independently tested and share your findings.

The most efficient and cost-effective solution, and environmentally sustainable option, is to install a quality water filter in your home and fill reusable bottles to take with you. There are a wide variety of filters available to suit your needs—whether fully installed or bench-top options (refrigerator filters are not very efficient at removing chemicals). And always ensure that you replace filters as per the manufacturer's specifications. Water bottles should ideally be made of glass or highest food-grade stainless steel. There are also plastic varieties available, but ensure these are BPA-free and never wash them in hot water, as heat accelerates plastic degeneration. Also discard bottles after six months of use, as all plastic deteriorates over time. The bottles can be recycled. Until such time as you find a suitable water filter, there are cask options available at most supermarkets.

How much water do we need?

You'll often hear "drink eight glasses of water a day." Our water needs vary from person to person and according to level of activity, exercise, temperature, humidity, age, and overall health. A widely accepted calculation for basic water need is forty millilitres of water per kilogram of body weight. For example, if you weigh 60 kilograms, your body needs 2.4 litres of water. Don't panic. This may seem like a lot of water, but you also get fluids from whole foods and caffeine-free teas (green tea contains caffeine and should be limited to one or two cups per day). In clinic, I find that most people aren't drinking enough water. So, if this includes you, start by increasing your intake gradually by one extra glass every few days. Persevere until you achieve your goal intake—the frequent visits to the toilet will cease once your body is fully hydrated.

Water is best consumed at room temperature, not cold and definitely not iced, as this affects absorption and your core temperature. Traditional Chinese medicine recommends that all fluids be consumed warm and never cold. It is further advised not to drink water with meals, as this can impair digestion. Sip water throughout the day. Use bottles or a jug for easy monitoring—it helps to have a visual gauge of how much you have, or haven't, consumed.

One common excuse I hear is, "I don't like water." Well, if you are drinking tap water, I don't blame you—it tastes disgusting. Clean water tastes delicious. However, if you feel you need a little flavour, try adding a few fresh mint leaves, freshly chopped ginger, or cucumber slices. Don't add lemon to a large amount of water (bottle or jug), as your dentist won't be happy at your next check-up—lemon juice in water sipped over a prolonged period can erode tooth enamel. Have some lemon juice in small amounts of water, preferably before a meal (helps digestion) and then rinse your mouth with clean water to prevent any damage to teeth.

I also often hear, "But I'm not thirsty." If you aren't consuming enough water, lack of thirst can be the result of dehydration. Start drinking water, and your thirst response will kick in. Caffeinated drinks, including coffee, tea, cola, and energy drinks, will dramatically increase your water needs. Otto Warburg, Nobel Prize-winner for medicine, stated, "One glass of Coca-Cola takes 32 glasses of water at pH of 10 to counteract the acid that the cola produces in our bodies." In other words, not all liquids provide hydration.

Water is not only essential for every single cell in your body. It also helps flush out toxins—whether metabolic or environmental—so start enjoying this wondrous life-giving clear liquid.

***

- ❖ Invest in a quality water filter.
- ❖ Drink forty millilitres of water per kilogram of body weight.

10
Final Steps of Preparation

> Before anything else, preparation is the key to success.
> —Alexander Graham Bell

Now that we have covered the fundamentals of preparation for a healthy baby, it's time to consider conception and pregnancy.

But before you do, it is wise for both the mother-to-be and father-to-be to have comprehensive blood pathology done through your health practitioner. In addition to being a valuable tool for assessing overall health, for the woman it is important to establish a baseline so any changes can be monitored throughout gestation. Recommended tests can be found in Appendix 3.

Other optional testing may include a hair tissue mineral analysis to assess your mineral levels and the presence of any heavy metals. This is an easy, non-invasive test using a hair sample, which usually provides results within two weeks. Ideally this should be included at the very beginning of your preparation to allow sufficient time for adequate toxin clearance and replenishment of nutrients.

If you have been trying to conceive for some time, if you experience menstrual issues, or if you have been diagnosed with or suspect you may have endometriosis or PCOS, then perhaps a hormone assessment may identify underlying factors. Blood hormone levels fluctuate and are only an approximate indication. Also, blood tests do not differentiate between the different forms of oestrogen (there are three). Appendix 3 lists functional laboratories where you can select from very comprehensive assessments that include hormone levels, as well as how your body processes these, to less costly options that will provide details of hormone levels only. My recommendation is the DUTCH Plus, which has been described as "the most comprehensive assessment for adrenal and sex hormones available in one test, which means more accurate diagnoses and more effective treatments." There are several options, so check with your naturopath which one best suits your needs. Hormone tests are also available for men. Should there be any questions surrounding genetic or hereditary conditions or if you have been exposed to a lot of chemicals and toxins, then investing in a DNA test may be advisable. Unfortunately, sometimes we just do not know how what we have been exposed to can affect our children. As an example, a young mother who used to work in a petrol station part-time and who was unaware of the importance of methylation and prenatal supplementation had a child with Down's syndrome. Fortunately, once she'd learned about how supplements can aid this condition and prevent future babies suffering a similar fate, her second child was born healthy. Various companies offer DNA tests. I've listed one in Appendix 3. But you can choose whichever you prefer. Please note that, to identify what SNPs you actually have, always request the raw data. This can then be interpreted by other organisations or a trained practitioner. Knowing what SNPs you have may help prevent complications or significant hormonal swings once your baby is born.

***

- ❖ Check for toxins in your body with an HTMA or functional pathology test.
- ❖ Check hormones and metabolism if appropriate.
- ❖ Check your DNA.

SECTION II
Conception

The basic fact is simple: life begins,
not at birth, but conception
—Ashley Montague

11

Ready for Conception

> The most important thing in life is knowing the most
> important things in life.
> —David F. Jackielo

Now that you know how to avoid environmental toxins, have cleaned up your body, and have incorporated a healthy wholefoods diet, you are ready to conceive. Congratulations for being committed and doing the oh-so-important preparation. This section will focus more on the mother's health as it relates to gestation, while men or partner take on more of a supportive role.

I also encourage you to re-read chapter 3, "Sperm Meets Egg?" just to reinforce the importance of having all nutrients available in your body at all times before conception and throughout pregnancy.

Blood pathology and other tests

Regular blood pathology is usually carried out by your consulting GP or obstetrician. In Australia, doctors usually recommend that pregnant women undertake a glucose tolerance test to assess for gestational diabetes. Many women report that this test is very unpleasant. There have been no reported increases in gestational diabetes diagnoses since this test was introduced. Discuss other options to assess your body's blood sugar levels and any possible tendency towards developing gestational diabetes with your doctor. Other options include HbA1c (haemoglobin A1C and fasting insulin assessment.

It is also a good idea to ensure your doctor checks your full thyroid profile prior to conception, each trimester during pregnancy, and a few months post birth.[94] Iodine levels should also be assessed prior to conception—this is usually done via urine, and your practitioner will be able to advise whether your levels are adequate or not. There is more information on the importance of iodine in the following chapter.

Some of the other recommended tests include checking iron levels, which should be optimal prior to conception due to the increased demand throughout pregnancy. A comprehensive list of tests and explanations can be found in Appendix 3.

12

Nutrition for Mother and Baby

> Those who think they have no time for healthy eating will sooner or later have to find time for illness.
> —Edward Stanley

Maternal and neonatal health outcomes are significantly influenced by nutrient availability throughout preconception, pregnancy, and lactation. Inadequate nutrition during preconception and pregnancy poses significant risks to the foetus, including impaired development, preterm birth, and low birth weight.[95] The first thousand days of life, starting from conception, represent a critical window of growth and development. Science and research continue to identify how everything in these early days affects your child in multiple ways, including their experiences, environment, and diet, as well as the mother's health and lifestyle during pregnancy. Most fascinating, however, is that, starting from conception, the foetus is actively responding to changes in the environment, using cues provided by the mother's physical and mental state to "predict" the kind of world they will be born into and altering their bodily structures accordingly.[96]

Maternal nutrient levels and overall health have a significant impact on the health and genetic expression of generations to come, thereby setting up the infant with the greatest potential for lifelong health. This relies on having a solid foundation of nutrients and omega-3 essential fats and a healthy gut microbiome. Hopefully, you have been diligent and prepared your body by nurturing it with all the healthy foods described in section I. Pregnant women require a varied diet and nutrient intake to accommodate increased needs during pregnancy and for the development and growth of a healthy baby.[97] Providing key nutrients lays a solid nutritional foundation for a healthy pregnancy and, most importantly, a healthy child. Most nutrients have multiple mechanisms of action and support various aspects of health.

The recommended total calorie intake of the macronutrients in a healthy diet for pregnant women is 20 per cent protein, 50 per cent carbohydrates, and 30 per cent fats. However, when you look at your plate, it is perhaps easier to imagine a quarter of your plate is protein; a quarter is starches like potatoes, sweet potatoes, pumpkin, or a healthy grain; and a half is vegetables and/or salad.

All the information outlined in chapter 5, "Diet," still applies throughout pregnancy and beyond. However, there are a few nutrients and specific foods that warrant special mention.

Vitamin D

Emerging research suggests vitamin D deficiency during prenatal development may increase the risk of several diseases, including multiple sclerosis, schizophrenia, type 1 diabetes, and cancer. The research clearly supports vitamin D in its involvement in foetal development, especially the brain and immune system. Maternal vitamin D insufficiency during pregnancy is significantly associated with offspring language impairment. Supplementation during pregnancy may reduce the risk of developmental language difficulties.[98]

Safe sun exposure on a regular basis is the most natural source of vitamin D, while dietary sources include fatty fish liver oils, butter, eggs, whole milk, and sprouted seeds. Blood tests will reveal if you need to supplement with vitamin D. Optimum levels of 25 OHD are between 100-200nmol/L. If so, always source a quality product (preferably oil in a capsule or drops) and keep it refrigerated.

Bone health

Skeletal health in neonates is dependent on the availability of key nutrients during foetal development throughout gestation. Adequate maternal levels of vitamin D are vital for offspring bone development.[99] Vitamin K is also a key factor required for the formation of the neonatal skeleton, as it promotes bone growth, prevents tissue calcification, and limits calcium reabsorption from bone.[100] Vitamin K is produced by a healthy gut microbiome. Dietary sources include animal products, vegetables, and some dairy. Lastly, manganese is an essential cofactor in bone formation.[101]

This is due to its role in the synthesis of chondroitin sulphate, which aids skeletal development by supporting the structural growth of bone tissue. Other nutrients essential for bone health are protein—for collagen production—and minerals, especially calcium. If you have been prescribed a calcium supplement, it is important to ensure that the body's pH or acid-alkaline state is balanced. In an acidic environment, excess calcium is dropped into blood, leading to plaque build-up. The form of calcium is also important—avoid calcium carbonate, as it is extremely difficult to break down and digest, often resulting in calcification of soft tissues like blood vessels and kidneys. Calcium phosphate, which correlates with the biochemical form in bones, is most readily absorbed. A hair tissue mineral analysis will help identify any nutrient deficiencies.

Minerals

Minerals are essential components of some tissues but also act as co-factors in hundreds of biochemical reactions in each cell of your body. There is an intricate relationship between minerals and toxins, like heavy metals. You will find more information on minerals and vitamins, functions, and food sources in Appendix 2. But a few deserve special mention here.

Iodine

Iodine supports maternal thyroid function during pregnancy and lactation due to its role in the production of thyroid hormones—free thyroxine (fT4) and triiodothyronine (fT3). Demand for iodine is increased during pregnancy, as the foetus is reliant on maternal T4, which is directly responsible for baby's cellular metabolism, nerve/brain development, and myelination during gestation.[102] Iodine deficiency in pregnancy is the leading preventable cause of intellectual impairment in the world. Due to iodine's role in foetal brain and nervous system development, a deficiency during pregnancy may lead to *irreversible damage*. Even mild iodine deficiency could prevent children and adolescents from attaining their full intellectual potential, leading to neurodevelopmental issues and increased risk of ADD.[103]

In Australia, 70 per cent of women of childbearing age are iodine deficient. All pregnant and lactating women should discuss iodine supplementation with a qualified natural health practitioner. It is essential to check your iodine levels before conception and also to check your thyroid's capacity to function properly throughout pregnancy—refer to Appendix 3 for tests. Iodine is an essential mineral that is critical for growth and development. Insufficient iodine status leads to goitre in adults and cretinism in infants, making this mineral particularly important for pregnant women. Iodine deficiency is a growing issue in Australia, largely due to depleted soils and recent changes in dairy sanitation practices, where the use of iodine for sterilisation has been replaced with chlorine.[104]

So, why are we so iodine deficient? In addition to poor soil quality, there are a few minerals that block iodine—fluoride, chlorine, and bromide. Fluoride (the industrial kind) and chlorine are added to the drinking water in many cities throughout the world. In warmer climates, swimming pools are also a source of chlorine—remember that our skin absorbs chemicals, and this includes chlorine. Bromide is an additive found in baked goods and many soft drinks. Please do not take iodine without first assessing your needs. The best form of this mineral is potassium iodide with iodine.

Iron

Your iron needs increase during pregnancy but particularly during the second trimester. Low iron is often associated with fatigue, especially during pregnancy. Prenatal iron intake has been shown to improve neurological outcomes in children, highlighting the importance of maternal iron adequacy.[105] Recommended amount of iron intake daily is ten to fifteen milligrams and up to thirty milligrams per day during pregnancy and lactation.[106] Iron is a mineral that is widely available in foods. It can be found in meat, raw parsley, poultry, eggs, organic tofu, nuts, seeds, whole grains, and green leafy vegetables. Iron is an essential part of haemoglobin—the red colouring agent of blood that transports oxygen through our body. Furthermore, iron is an essential mineral used in many biochemical reactions in our body and is widely distributed in many tissues, not only the blood.

Dairy products can reduce iron absorption, as can tea consumption—both black and green teas contain tannins, which bind iron, so it's best not to have any tea with or within an hour of meals. Vitamin D and calcium supplements should be taken away from iron. Any gut issues such as inflammation, coeliac disease, or irritable bowel syndrome can also negatively influence iron absorption. Avoid coffee with or within an hour of meals, as it also impacts iron nutrient absorption. Ways to improve iron absorption include having colourful vegies or salads with meals (capsicum, beetroot, spinach, and other green leafy vegetables) or consuming bitter vegetables or fruit before or during the meal to increase the flow of stomach acid.

Having good levels of stomach acid is essential for proper iron utilisation; otherwise, intestinal absorption is compromised. Minerals such as sodium and potassium may improve iron absorption in the body, as will vitamin C and B-group. Toxic metals such as mercury, cadmium, lead, and aluminium will compete with iron absorption, so it's essential to ensure these metals are reduced or non-existent for effective iron metabolism. Some medications and drugs affect iron absorption or metabolism, including antacids, aspirin, indomethacin, methyldopa, neomycin, tetracycline, and penicillamine. So does excess intake of some minerals (so don't self-prescribe).

If taking an iron supplement, it is best to take it every second day, as this aids absorption.[107] Ferrous fumarate or iron polymaltose are frequently prescribed to replete body iron stores.[108] However, the high doses required cause numerous undesirable side effects, including gastrointestinal upset, increased oxidative stress, subclinical inflammation, and gut microbiome alterations. Lactoferrin, which is an iron-binding protein, is an essential regulator of iron homeostasis, as it increases iron absorption, reduces inflammation, and sequesters iron during infection.[109] Another beneficial form is iron glycinate.

To avoid the need for an iron infusion during pregnancy, it's best to ensure your levels are adequate prior to conception. However, if your doctor prescribes an iron infusion during pregnancy, it's best to take additional vitamin C and other antioxidants in the week leading up to and for at least three weeks post infusion to offset oxidative damage. Use a quality vitamin C powder, which is buffered (that is, not acidic) and contains other supportive antioxidants such as beta-carotene, vitamin E, zinc, rutoside, hesperidin, CoQ10, and alpha lipoic acid. Taking smaller, more frequent doses will be of greater benefit than taking a heaped teaspoon once a day.

Exercise

I often get asked, "Can I continue to exercise when pregnant?" It is always best to discuss exercise with your obstetrician. But generally, if you have been exercising regularly well prior to conception, the response is yes.

Movement is always beneficial and should be amended to suit your capabilities, energy levels, and physical size—as your tummy grows, you may need to find new forms of exercise. Antenatal yoga, water-based gentle exercises, or simply going for a pleasant walk in nature will all support your fitness and overall health without placing too much stress on you or your baby. Restricting exercise to less than forty-five minutes is recommended to prevent episodes of low blood sugar.[110]

Neural tube defects

Gestational neurodevelopment is highly sensitive to nutritional status. Insufficient nutrient availability, high levels of oxidative stress, and poor blood sugar control may elevate the risk of neural tube defects (NTDs).[111] Choline and vitamins B6 and B12 have been demonstrated to lower the risk of NTDs in pregnancy when combined with adequate folic acid.[112] A large body of evidence supports the use of folic acid in lowering NTD risk—shown to reduce incidence by a significant 50 per cent to 75 per cent.[113] Due to food fortification and over-supplementation with the inactive form of folate, there has been a rise in MTHFR polymorphisms over the past few decades. You might like to refer back to the chapter on methylation. If you have been diagnosed with one of the MTHFR SNPs, taking calcium folinate, 5-methyl tetrahydrofolate or levomefolate (activated forms) may be more beneficial for you, as these can directly enter the methylation cycle.[114]

Choline is an often-deficient essential nutrient needed by the developing brain as a precursor of acetylcholine.[115] This key neurotransmitter regulates nerve tissue and brain formation.[116] Choline is also a key component of methyl groups. Lutein, which makes up 59 per cent of total brain carotenoids, is found in high concentrations within the infant nervous system, particularly in those parts of the brain involved in learning and memory.[117] Foods sources of lutein include yellow and green fruit and vegetables like capsicums, carrots, pumpkin, sweet potato, tomatoes, green leafy vegetables, parsley, and eggs. Providing these important nutrients can help support neural growth and healthy brain development.

Maternal microbiome

The maternal microbiome is instrumental in the development of the infant microbiome, with the transfer of organisms affecting a wide range of organ systems beyond the gastrointestinal tract. Probiotic supplementation during pregnancy may beneficially influence both the maternal and infant gastrointestinal microbiota, and impact clinical outcomes. For example, if the mother supplements with specific strains of probiotics during pregnancy and lactation, the risk of children developing allergy-based conditions such as eczema or receiving behavioural-based diagnoses, including for attention deficit hyperactivity disorder (ADHD), can be reduced, particularly in those cases where there is a family history of atopic conditions. Gut dysbiosis can lead to vaginal dysbiosis characterised by insufficient lactobacillus strains, which has been linked with increased risk of miscarriage.[118] Refer back to the chapter on gut health to refresh your memory as to how important this is and always consult a qualified natural health professional before taking any supplements, including a probiotic.

***

- ❖ The first one thousand days of life, starting from conception, represent a critical window of growth and development.
- ❖ Due to iodine's role in foetal brain and nervous system development, a deficiency during pregnancy may lead to irreversible damage.
- ❖ Gut dysbiosis can lead to vaginal dysbiosis, which has been linked with increased risk of miscarriage.

13

Pregnancy Woes

> Pregnancy is a process that invites you to surrender to the unseen force behind all life.
> —Judy Ford

Morning sickness

Major causes of morning sickness include lack of sleep, poor liver function, toxicity, and blood sugar level imbalances. If your liver is struggling with the added hormones of early pregnancy, it can cause nausea and vomiting. There's not much that can be done about toxins once you're pregnant other than avoiding further exposure. One way of supporting good blood sugar levels is to have a thick protein smoothie first thing in the morning or aim to have your largest meal early in the day. Once pregnant, only take anti-nausea support that has been clinically trialled and shown to be completely safe. Thalidomide comes to mind here, as it was claimed safe, only to be linked with severe physical damage to babies born to mothers who took the drug. There are some traditional Chinese herbs (prescribed by a qualified practitioner) that can be very beneficial and safe in relieving morning sickness, as can acupuncture.

At the first sign of discomfort, ensure that you are not dehydrated—make sure you are drinking enough water (40 ml/kg body weight. Sipping water can help relieve nausea, heartburn, acidity, and indigestion. You can add a little lemon juice or fresh ginger to a glass of water or try adding one teaspoon of bicarbonate soda—sip slowly until reflux stops (usually ten to fifteen minutes). Sometimes, slowly chewing on some plain bread before getting up can lessen nausea and prevent vomiting. Review your diet—are you eating enough protein?

Vitamin B6 administered within the first trimester of pregnancy has been shown to improve symptom severity if levels were deficient. In a randomised, controlled trial, vitamin B6 was shown to be as effective as ginger and more efficacious than placebo in reducing the severity of morning sickness using a validated screening tool. However, you should ideally be supplementing with a quality B complex product, which would contain B6. Always tell your health practitioner if you are already taking any other supplements, as too much vitamin B6 can cause nerve irritation.

Zinc is another essential mineral that, when lacking, can also contribute to morning sickness. If you are unable to tolerate oral supplements, ask your health care professional to prescribe compounded skin creams.

There is an upside to the constant nausea and vomiting—morning sickness is associated with a decreased risk of miscarriage.

Some women experience morning sickness to the extreme—this is known as hyperemesis gravidarum. I have seen a few women in my clinic who had experienced hyperemesis with previous pregnancies (before they came to see me). Believe me when I say that this is not a pleasant way to spend nearly nine months. While there are medical treatments to stop the vomiting, I am always concerned about possible consequences to the baby's health. Looking at this from a holistic perspective, we must consider the liver and other lifestyle factors. The women I saw experienced significant relief after receiving homeopathic liver support. They were then able to enjoy their pregnancy, rather than being bedridden with a bucket next to them. To prevent hyperemesis, I would very strongly recommend following the recommendations at the beginning of this book, especially as they relate to environmental toxins. The cleaner your body is prior to conception, the easier it will cope with pregnancy.

Dehydration

Especially during extended periods of morning sickness accompanied by vomiting, dehydration can occur. If you are struggling to keep water down, try adding some mineral citrates (magnesium, potassium, sodium) to help replace lost electrolytes. Mineral tissue salts can also be helpful, especially if your stomach acid levels are low following bouts of vomiting.

Symptoms of dehydration can include headaches, nausea, cramps, swelling of hands and feet, and dizziness. It is particularly important to ensure good hydration in the third trimester, as dehydration can trigger contractions and preterm labour. Drinking sufficient water also helps prevent urinary tract infections, which can be common during pregnancy.

Pregnancy and the gall bladder

Gall stones can form at any age and occur in both men and women. Over 6.3 million females and 14.2 million males in the United States between the ages of twenty and seventy-four have gallstones.[119] Pregnancy also plays a role in the formation of gall stones, as higher levels of progesterone decrease gall bladder contractability, which can lead to stone formation. Bitter foods like radicchio, chicory, dandelion leaves, silver beet, and grapefruit all support bile flow. Dandelion tea is a gentle and effective bitter available from most supermarkets or health food stores and a great alternative to coffee.

Warming spices in the diet can improve sluggish digestion and aid in relieving nausea, dyspepsia (belching), and indigestion. Ginger, cardamom, cumin, and coriander are beneficial, in particular grated fresh ginger brewed into a tea can help relieve nausea. Sour foods also aid digestion, and adding the juice of half a fresh lemon to a small quantity of water, especially consumed before meals helps support stomach acid levels. Other sour foods include kimchi, sauerkraut, mustard greens, guava, rhubarb, pomegranate, and pickles. Good levels of stomach acid are required to trigger the release of bile from the gall bladder, thereby helping prevent stone formation.

Bile is actually produced by the liver. And to help ensure that it is produced properly, flows well, and does not form stones, liver support is essential. This brings us back to the preparation phase and supporting liver and gut health.

Baby brain

As already mentioned in the chapter on essential fatty acids, DHA supports brain health and function. As your baby grows inside you, its demand on nutrients increases. There may be times throughout gestation when you feel unable to think clearly. Some pregnant ladies have described it as "not being able to string two words together." During these phases, increase your EPA/DHA supplements. If you are taking one or two capsules once daily, take them twice or even three times daily, until your brain function returns. And it will. You may also need to increase your prenatal multivitamin for several days. Check your diet to ensure you are getting all the recommended nutrients.

Stretch marks

Daily massage of the abdomen, hips, thighs, buttocks, and breasts is advised to help keep skin pliable and able to stretch. This is a wonderfully nurturing activity to share with your partner. There are some great products available that are free from nasties—but check the label and make sure the product does not contain any petrochemicals. Oils to use either alone or as a blend of a few include coconut, sweet almond, apricot kernel, avocado, rosehip, jojoba, Mongolian sea-buckthorn, calendula, or argan. You can also add a few drops of pure essential oils of mandarin and some natural vitamin E. Use between five and ten drops of pure essential to twenty millilitres of carrier oil. During pregnancy, no other essential oils are deemed safe.

Stretch marks occur due to tearing of the skin tissue, most often due to sudden expansion or sudden weight loss (after birth). A lack of zinc can make skin more prone to tearing, so ensure your levels are adequate well before you fall pregnant—it all goes back to good prevention practices.

Pre-eclampsia

A rise in blood pressure (hypertension) accompanied by fluid retention and loss of proteins in urine may be indicators of pre-eclampsia. This condition occurs mostly after week twenty of gestation and can lead to damage of the blood vessels in organs such as the brain, liver, lungs, and kidneys. If left untreated, it can lead to organ failure, requiring immediate delivery of the baby. Research has identified risk factors for pre-eclampsia, which include nutrient deficiencies (especially vitamin

B12), low antioxidant levels, obesity, diabetes, age over forty, stress, insulin resistance, hypothyroidism, IVF, pre-existing renal disease, and hypertension.

In a large study of pregnant women, diet was again identified as both contributor and remedy, with those consuming a high vegetable / plant food-based diet and EFA oils showing a 28 per cent reduced risk of pre-eclampsia. A diet high in processed foods including processed meats, salty snacks, and sweet drinks led to 21 per cent increased risk.[120] Specific nutritional deficiencies increasing risk of pre-eclampsia include low DHA, magnesium, iodine, calcium, and especially vitamin D deficiency, which heightens risk by 540 per cent.[121]

Allergies and atopy

Questions that frequently get asked by mums-to-be include whether they should avoid certain foods during pregnancy. In particular, any foods that cause them distress. If there is an allergic response to any foods, these should definitely be avoided, as the IgE antibodies can cross the placenta and may prime the foetal immune system for later reactivity. If there is a history of atopy in the family—asthma and/or eczema—then I would suggest you follow the recommendations relating to toxin exposure and diet in the first section of this book. Even if you cannot completely prevent allergy or atopy in your baby, you will know you have done all you can to at least minimise any reactions in the future.

Foods that cause distress are not necessarily triggering an allergic response—reactions can reflect gut and microbiome imbalances. Review the section on gut health, as this usually alleviates any food-related reactions. Being able to eat a wide variety of foods is the foundation of good nutrition. You will find more information about eczema in section III.

***

- ❖ Dedicated preparation, including removal of toxins, may help prevent unpleasant symptoms during pregnancy.
- ❖ Ensure good nutrient levels and supplement if needed.

14

Preparing for Birth

> When you change the way you view birth, the way you
> birth will change.
> —Marie Mongan

We are fortunate here in Australia to have options when it comes to birthing a baby—whether you choose to have your baby in a hospital environment, at a birth centre, or at home, it should be your decision and that of your partner. You'll most likely find that everyone you meet, especially family and friends, all have some advice for you. Remember that this advice usually comes from a place of concern for you, so if it all gets a bit much at times, just smile and say, "Thank you." Advice can be about the birth, the best way to feed your baby—breast or bottle—sleeping, using a dummy, and things you perhaps never thought of.

I'd like to share with you two births that were totally different. The first is the birth of my first daughter. My pregnancy had gone incredibly smoothly. I felt great, and all was proceeding well according to my doctors. You can imagine how surprised my husband I were when, at thirty-one weeks, my waters suddenly broke. Off to the nearest clinic we went—nearly an hour away along winding, partly gravel roads, as we were living on a rural property at the time. Then, after a jab in the arm to stop contractions, I was bundled into an ambulance and taken to the nearest larger hospital on a two-hour night-time dash. After five days' strict bed-rest (you have no idea how wonderful a shower is until you are told you can't have one), it was time.

My daughter was born by emergency Caesarean section and spent her first eighteen hours in a humidicrib. Fortunately, her lungs were developed, and I could hold her the following day, although I was heavily sedated with morphine due to the extreme surgery I'd had. As she'd been early, my daughter's sucking reflex had not developed, and feeding was almost impossible. Weight loss followed, and what little milk I had soon stopped.

Great nursing staff and perseverance for the next four weeks got her strong enough to bring home, where a strict feeding and monitoring regimen had to be adhered to. We were blessed that she was so strong. And by the time she reached her expected full term, she weighed just over nine pounds. When my daughter and her husband were expecting their first child, they decided on a home water birth, with midwife and doula present. You'd be excused in thinking I may have voiced concerns following my experience, but I knew they had done their research and taken the time to prepare for labour and birth. The birth was peaceful, in their own home, with the support of capable professionals. It was indeed a very beautiful experience for all concerned. So, you see, there are options—you just need to do your research and listen to your own body. My daughter knew this was the right decision for her and her baby.

We often hear that women have been giving birth for centuries—which is true. But we are all different. I like to encourage women to get in tune with the baby growing inside them. There is and always will be a bond that cannot be explained or described. Listen to that bond and follow your instincts. Firstborn babies are notorious for going over the expected term for delivery, so provided you are both well and being monitored by medical professionals, don't worry if your little one is in no hurry to be born.

For the final trimester of your pregnancy, I recommend taking a herbal tonic prescribed by your naturopath/herbalist to help strengthen the uterus muscles, which will aid in the birthing process as well as passing the placenta. There are also essential oils that, when massaged into the lower back, can help relieve birthing discomfort and support the process. These include clary sage, neroli, and jasmine, with myrrh beneficial in assisting during a prolonged, difficult labour. These should be in a carrier oil such as jojoba, sweet almond, or even olive oil using a maximum of ten drops total essential oil to twenty-five millilitres of carrier oil. Some essential oils also help breast milk to flow and can be used during any congestion in the breasts and to help prevent mastitis—fennel, aniseed, and jasmine in jojoba oil (avoid the nipple region when applying these oils). Essential oils are medicinal, and only pure quality oils should be used—if in doubt, seek the advice of a qualified aromatherapist.

Throughout pregnancy, your body is accommodating the growing foetus. To avoid any physical discomfort—back, hip, or leg pain—I highly recommend seeing a qualified chiropractor or osteopath to keep your body aligned and aid the birthing process. As the body prepares for birth, your joints and ligaments become more pliable and elastic. When your baby prepares to be born, it will seek out the most comfortable position. I'd like to share Erin's experience; she had done everything to prepare for conception and had enjoyed a pleasant pregnancy. But when the time came for birth, her pelvis was too tight, resulting in the baby moving into a breach position. An emergency caesarean section followed, associated with significant trauma, as she had been in labour for several hours. Fortunately, neither Erin nor her son sustained any lasting problems, and she has gone on to have another healthy boy.

Complementary therapies can be highly beneficial in supporting both pregnancy and the birthing process. So don't discount acupuncture, aromatherapy, naturopathy, homeopathy, massage, and chiropractic or osteopathic/cranio-sacral therapy.

The placenta

There are varying cultural traditions relating to the placenta—in some cultures, women eat the placenta, believing it will provide concentrated nutrients. In others, the placenta is dehydrated and turned into capsules or a tonic. Other mothers prefer to allow the placenta to fall off by itself, enabling the baby to get the benefit of all the remaining nutrients it contains. Whatever your personal choice, I would recommend assessing the placenta for possible toxins prior to any consumption. Recall the information under environmental toxins relating to how these are concentrated in the placenta. Even if you do not wish to consume the placenta, having it assessed thoroughly for toxins may be helpful in knowing what your newborn baby has been exposed to. Knowledge is power when it comes to preventing or alleviating any possible negative health outcomes.

Homeopathy

Something many of my new mums and dads found extremely helpful was consulting a qualified homeopath prior to the birth of their baby. They were able to learn about remedies and how to use these in case their bub got any unpleasant symptoms, including fever, skin irritation, or colic. They also learned about prophylactic options to protect against common childhood diseases. Homeopathic first aid kits are a valuable asset to have in your home medicine cabinet.

***

- ❖ Each birth is unique.
- ❖ Research your options and choose what is best for you and your baby.
- ❖ Always have a back-up plan.

SECTION III
Birth

Three things remain with us from Paradise: stars, flowers and children.
—Dante Alighieri

15

Congratulations on Your New Baby

A baby is something you carry inside you for nine months, in your arms for three years and in your heart until the day you die
—Mary Mason

What would be the one most important piece of advice I would give a mother following the birth? *Remember to look after yourself.* I've seen many new mums in my clinic, and their sole focus is their beautiful newborn baby (totally understandable—but not to the detriment of your own health. You need good, nutritious food and sleep, so try and rest whenever your baby is sleeping. I get it. You just want to hold this precious bundle all the time and never put your little one down. Whether or not you are breastfeeding, your body needs nutrients to help it return to pre-baby strength.

Breast or formula?

You may have already decided on your preferred feeding method—breast or formula or a combination of both. You may have had your heart set on breastfeeding, only to find that this was not an option for you. It happens—it happened to me. Do your research and select a quality organic formula. There are many options available these days—including whey (dairy), goat, and camel milk. Don't laugh—camel milk is the closest to human breast milk. If bubs can't tolerate one brand, try others until you find one that is suitable for your baby. Perhaps the most important consideration when bottle-feeding is to *never* use unfiltered tap water to prepare the formula. The levels of chlorine, fluoride, and other chemicals are highly toxic for such a small body ill-equipped to detox these substances.

Constipation can often occur when using formula. Change brands or give a little tepid purified water in case of dehydration (especially in hot weather). Sometimes, a very gentle tummy massage (really just gentle stroking) can get things moving. Using only the flat tips of your fingers, with baby lying on its back, start in the lower right side of the abdomen around the hip bone, gently stroke up towards the ribs, move across under the ribs, then down to baby's left side. Repeat. You may notice your baby relaxing and enjoying this very gentle massage. Homeopathic suppositories are an effective and safe option if your little one is very constipated.

Breastfeeding is convenient, as there are no bottles to sterilise or milk to warm up—breast milk is always there, on demand and in tune with your baby's needs. It helps give your baby antibodies for immune health and microbiome for digestive health. It can also be useful for little irritations, including sore eyes—the natural antimicrobial effect of breast milk can quickly soothe and clear conjunctivitis. It is one of the reasons many mums freeze their breast milk for later medicinal use.

If you do decide to breastfeed, remember to drink sufficient purified water (to help milk flow) and eat a very healthy diet to ensure your baby receives all the nutrients it needs. If your milk is not flowing freely or your baby appears to be constantly demanding more, try drinking aniseed tea. Recent research identified that consuming two grams of dried aniseed as a tea—combined with other herbal tea if you prefer—three times a day increased both milk flow and quality. Foods that support milk flow include lettuce, basil, dill, fenugreek, carrot juice, spinach, sesame, and fennel.[122] Also bear in mind that, if your baby displays signs of tummy upset, colic, or vomiting (especially projectile) or just long periods of being unsettled and crying, look at what you have been eating. Interestingly, aniseed, fennel, and fenugreek are also known to soothe a baby's upset tummy. Read about Natalie's experience in the next section.

With social media and opinions freely given, one thing you need to remember is that, whether or not you breastfeed your baby, it is your choice, and you should never feel guilty about your choice.

Colic, reflux, and tears

What do you do if your baby is just not happy? What if he or she won't stop crying even when you have checked all the obvious—dry nappy, fed and burped, warm/cool enough, comfortable? What if, after feeding, the milk comes back as a projectile?

I'd like to share the experience Natalie had when she brought her firstborn son home from hospital. A boy who had been happy at birth developed undiagnosed colic and reflux, with incessant crying. Severe sleep deprivation, frustration, and rising stress levels followed in what Natalie describes as "one of the toughest most brutal stages of my life."[123] This stage would continue for most of her son's first year, with doctors declaring he was fine and would grow out of it. Natalie was what you would consider a healthy attentive mum, breastfeeding with great milk supply. So, what was wrong?

When breastfeeding your baby, everything you eat and are exposed to passes through the milk. This can affect your baby—as it did Natalie's little boy.

Look at your diet. Two of the most frequent causes of colic and reflux in babies are dairy and wheat. Some babies just cannot metabolise certain proteins from these foods. Eliminate dairy first, and if the colic or reflux continue, then eliminate wheat as well. But before you go ahead and start eliminating any other foods, speak to a qualified naturopath or homeopath who has experience in infant care.

So, what was the outcome for Natalie? Fortunately, after nearly a year, she found a doctor who actually listened and suggested she try the bottle—which she did. Her son was immediately transformed into a happy baby. So, while breast is definitely best, it may just not be best for you and your baby. If you cannot breastfeed, for whatever reason or simply make the choice not to, never be bullied into feeling guilty.

For cases of incidental or mild colic, there are a few traditional options you may find helpful, such as a little fennel seed tea. If formula feeding, check ingredients, as these can be causing upset. Other options to help settle a distraught little one is a warm bath with a few drops of essential oils—during the first few weeks, the only oil recommended safe to use is German or blue chamomile. After two to three weeks, you can rotate oils, using lavender or mandarin in the bath-water. Oh, when it comes to bath-water, remember that regular tap water contains chlorine, fluoride, aluminium, and other nasties not suitable to immerse your newborn in. The skin is our largest organ, absorbing everything it is exposed to. We are back to water filters—it may be worth considering a whole-of-house filter or at least a detachable tap filter to ensure your precious new baby is bathing in clean water.

Other causes of colic and reflux may be linked to the actual birth process, especially if this was prolonged or involved any mechanical assistance (forceps). In this case, I recommend taking your baby to see an osteopath trained in cranio-sacral technique—an extremely gentle form of correcting misalignments of the cranium and spine. Please don't freak out—this type of therapy does not involve "cracking or crunching" the bones, and it can really turn your life around. And while you are there, have an adjustment yourself to put your body back into alignment following pregnancy and giving birth.

Baby's immune system

A newborn baby doesn't have an immune system yet, which is why colostrum and breast milk are so important. This begins the colonisation, along with a vaginal birth and introduction of enzymes. From the moment of birth, medical staff will be ready to administer a vitamin K injection and, in Australia, a hepatitis B vaccine. Two months later, the rigorous vaccination protocol begins. If you have any doubts or questions, please do your research and seek professional advice, as there may be other options to support your child's immune health.[124]

After all you have learned about antibiotic use and gut health, it would be wise to avoid giving your baby this type of medicine if possible. Here are a few words of advice from one of Australia's leading homeopathic doctors, Dr Isaac Golden: "Parents approach me regarding vaccine options for their infants, and for themselves leading up to the birth, as well as general immunisation for all ages for overseas travel. They also approach me (if they have vaccinated their child) regarding either general vaccine detoxing of a healthy child, or the treatment of vaccine injuries if there are clear symptoms following the vaccination. The above issues can be done by phone and email with people living anywhere in Australia."[125] There are, of course, other good homeopaths around who you could ask for advice as well.

***

- ❖ Breastfeed if you can.
- ❖ Choose a quality organic formula if breastfeeding is not an option.
- ❖ Never discount complementary therapies.

16

Time for Solid Food

> Investing in early childhood nutrition is a surefire strategy.
> The returns are incredibly high.
> —Anne M. Mulcahy[126]

Every baby is different, and each will be ready for solid food at a different age, which could range between three and six months. The same considerations apply to your baby as to you—avoid processed foods, select organic non-GMO produce as much as possible, and start with a little of one vegetable at a time. Introducing foods into baby's diet can be made easier by following a few simple suggestions:

- Avoid your bub being sensitised by the more common foods known to cause allergies, such as milk, wheat, soy, eggs, tomatoes, and citrus by leaving their introduction until the baby is a little older.
- Introduce foods one at a time so that any reactions can be identified.
- Reactions may reflect intolerance and not necessarily allergy. Signs may include hives; flash on the face, mouth, or buttocks; eczema; wheezing; runny nose; diarrhoea with increase in temperature; or being grizzly or unusually tired.
- When introducing a food, give the baby only one teaspoon the first day, followed by two teaspoons the second day and continue this way, gradually increasing the quantity until a full serving is taken. If baby rejects the food, stop that food for at least a week before trying a small quantity again.
- If a reaction occurs, immediately stop the offending food, and wait for one week before trying again or introducing any other new foods. A reaction does not necessarily mean it is causing an allergic response, just that your baby may not be ready or that the food contains chemicals.
- Keep a record of foods as they are introduced and any reactions for future reference.

- Tolerated foods may be combined at a later date.
- Where possible use organic produce to avoid ingestion of chemicals, pesticides, antibiotics, and hormones.
- Never add salt, sugar, yeast, or vegemite. These can lead to problems such as allergies or addictions later in life. Most adverse reactions are caused by wheat and dairy.

Food preparation

I have been asked to include some suggestions on how best to prepare the first few meals your baby will eat. As these should involve vegetables, it is best to begin with blander flavours and textures. Zucchini or squash are usually well received—these should be lightly steamed until just soft enough to mash. With softer vegetables, a fork may suffice. Or you can use a blender to puree until you achieve a softer, creamier consistency. Some babies are sensitive to textures so try both smooth and slightly chunkier consistencies. As your baby will likely only have a few mouthfuls during the initial phases, it is helpful to freeze any unused food into ice cube trays or incorporate that vegetable into adults' meal to avoid any waste. Any frozen food can be stored in glass containers and defrosted at room temperature for future use.

Please, never use a microwave oven to defrost, warm, or cook food for your baby. Microwaves affect the frequency of all cells, including water, which makes up most of our food (and our body).

To avoid your baby overdeveloping the sweet taste receptors on the tongue, alternate sweeter vegetables like carrots, sweet potatoes, and pumpkin with more savoury flavours. Once single vegetables are well tolerated, you can begin to combine different flavours and textures. The same tips apply if you choose baby-led-weaning to introduce solid foods. All these guidelines regarding food were unknown to me when I had my girls. Once milk wasn't enough for them, I'd boil some oats in water (much more water than needed to make porridge) and strain the oats, retaining the slightly gluggy watery residue. This served as a transition from milk to solids, at which time I'd blend the oats to a creamy consistency.

Thereafter, I'd simply blend the vegetables my husband and I were having for our meal and feed that to the girls. The only time I ever resorted to bought baby food was on our once-a-month shopping trip, which involved a three-hour round car trip, not including the time it took to do four weeks' worth of grocery shopping. Fortunately, they were both good eaters, but this varies from child to child.

A friend of mine has two beautiful boys—the older literally eats all different foods with gusto, whereas the younger boy limits his intake to only a few, very politely declining anything he considers unpalatable with a "no thank you, Mummy." She has learned to camouflage vegetables into his favourite foods—a tactic many mums learn to ensure their babies receive the nutrients they need.

Time frames for introducing solid foods to your baby

Vegetables

4–6 months — First try squash, carrots, spinach, sweet potatoes, cabbage, cauliflower, broccoli, turnips, eggplant, and pumpkin. Try to vary the colour, texture, and consistency of the foods. Lightly steam the vegetables and mash. Leave peas and beans until later, as these are harder to digest.

18 months — Tomatoes—start with low acid varieties.

24 months — Corn (organic).

Fruit

4–6 months — Try stewed pears, apricots, prunes, and then ripe mashed bananas, remembering these contain a lot of sugar and should not be given too often. Note that bananas may cause constipation.

12 months — Apples and peaches, raw fruit.

18 months — Citrus.

24 months — Berries.

Cereal/grains

6 months   Introduce a variety of single grains such, as porridge or oatmeal, barley, or rice. Do not mix the grains.

9 months   Other non-wheat varieties

Milk

The ideal milk for baby is breast milk until at least 12 months of age, or as long as you decide. This may be varied by the addition of filtered water from a cup at about 7 to 9 months. If supplementation is needed, watch for allergies as noted above. Milk is a food and should not be given as a drink. Avoid nut and oat milks, as these are generally low in nutrients and high in sugar and early over-consumption of nut-based milks may lead to intolerances later on.

Meat

6-9 months   Lamb, veal, and then beef and chicken—organic or grass-fed.

Fish

12 months   Start with non-oily white fleshed fish.

Eggs

12 months   Start by giving a quarter teaspoon of yolk only three times a week max. Then increase by half a teaspoon at a time until baby can eat the whole yolk without adverse symptoms. Once baby is used to the yolk, give very small amounts of egg white, gradually increasing as with the yolk.

Nuts

5 years — Nuts are dangerous for any child under the age of five years, as they can be inhaled and lead to choking. Nuts should always be given under close supervision. Pureed nuts in food or smooth nut butters may be given sooner, but always be aware of any possible allergies. Note that some cultures consume nuts from a very young age.

Chocolate/lollies

Avoid any products that contain artificial colours, flavours, or preservatives. Very small quantities of good quality chocolate may be given on the rare occasion after five years of age.

Soft drinks/sodas

Avoid all fizzy drinks and cordial, as these are laden with sugar, artificial sweeteners, colours, and flavourings, as well as preservatives. These are unnecessary, and purified water is always best. I definitely recommend you never give your child any soft drinks. A freshly pressed organic vegetable and fruit juice as an occasional healthy treat when they are older is fine.

I often get asked, "But what about treats?" My response is, "What do you mean by the word 'treat'?"

Ask your grandparents how often they had treats when they were growing up. It may have been an ice cream once a month or a few lollies. The problem we are faced with these days is that treats are becoming more of the norm, rather than something to be savoured on very rare, special occasions. A treat can be something that is nutritious—homemade baking where you control the ingredients (and quantity of sugar), rather than something store bought, which is full of ingredients with numbers. Treats do not need to be edible—a treat can be spending quality time together or creating special memories.

Oral health

When should you start brushing your baby's teeth? The answer is when the first tooth appears. It is never too early to start brushing your child's teeth, as this promotes good habits for later in life. Use either a very soft natural toothbrush or a finger brush to gently clean the teeth and gums. Do not use any toothpaste at this stage. This is just to get your baby used to the feeling of cleaning teeth. There is no need to use any toothpaste until your child is old enough to rinse its mouth well and spit out all residue. So, for the first year or two, just use filtered water and a soft brush to clean teeth after every meal. Dr Bill Kellner-Read's book *Toxic Bite—An Investigation into Truth Decay* is an excellent resource for your home library.

***

- ❖ Offer your child a variety of foods appropriate to age and culture.
- ❖ Be the mama/papa bear and teach your child which foods are acceptable and which are not.
- ❖ Even treats can be nutritious and beneficial.

17

Skin and Other Irritations

Skin is a reflection of internal health

Skin irritations can occur on any part of your baby's body and may include nappy rash, cradle cap, or eczema. As the skin is the largest organ of the body, it is often used to expel substances that cannot otherwise be cleared. A baby's body and internal detoxification organs are poorly developed, often leaving skin as the only option. For mosquito or insect stings, apply some fresh aloe vera gel to the site to remove the itch and accelerate healing. You'll need to get a plant—these are available from most garden supply nurseries—as the gel needs to be fresh rather than out of a jar.

Nappy rash or any form of redness or irritation around the bottom may be the result of acidic urine or faeces. Once again, look to diet—if breastfeeding, review what you have consumed for up to three days prior to any redness appearing on your baby's bottom. Some common foods that can cause acidity include oranges, mandarins, pineapple, tomatoes, and mango. But all babies are different, and it could be another food that triggers acidic urine or faeces. If formula feeding, perhaps include a few small feeds of purified water given throughout the day, as dehydration can also lead to over acidic urine.

To help soothe the inflamed regions, you can use organic coconut, calendula and/or rosehip oil as a carrier, adding a few drops of pure essential oils of lavender and German chamomile. Add two drops of essential oil to approximately one tablespoon or twenty millilitres of carrier oil. If there is a lot of heat, try some fresh aloe vera gel. Avoid using baby oil, as this is petroleum-based and impairs the skin's ability to release toxins.

Cradle cap is a condition often seen in newborn babies, where crusty or oily, scaly patches appear on the scalp. The condition is not painful or itchy, and the scales should not be picked at or removed. A contributing factor is gut imbalance due to poor microbiome as often occurs in babies born via Caesarean section and/or prematurely (my first daughter had cradle cap). If you are breastfeeding, ensure you are still taking your prenatal formula containing all the B complex vitamins and biotin, which is especially beneficial for cradle cap. You can also use a baby probiotic— mix a little powder with your breast milk and rub around baby's gums. Avoid using any chemicals or oils on the scalp.

For **eczema**, if you are breastfeeding look at your diet. Babies can react to foods that mum is eating. Check for the usual culprits—wheat and dairy—but also consider eggs, soy, and sugar. Here's the story of a mum seeking help for her three-week old daughter who had developed eczema. As allergies were widespread on both sides of her and her husband's family, she wanted to do all she could to spare her daughter from a lifetime of atopic illnesses. On the advice of her paediatrician, she eliminated eggs from her diet, and her daughter's eczema cleared up within a week. The mum continued to breastfeed for two years, seeking to give her daughter's immune system the best foundation for later in life. It worked—the daughter is now in her teens, and except for the occasional indulgence in known allergen-creating foods, her skin is fine. A further bonus is that she never developed asthma or hay fever, both of which are common in atopy. When it comes to skin irritations, we always look at gut health. The skin is our largest organ and is often used to clear toxins. Probiotics, in particular the strain *Lactobacillus rhamnosus* HN001, have been shown to reduce the symptoms of eczema during pregnancy and while breastfeeding.[127] *L. rhamnosus* was clinically tested, with results revealing significant reduction of symptoms up to age four. Interestingly, it also reduced the prevalence of rhino-conjunctivitis at four years of age.[128] The fact that supporting eczema with probiotics eased the condition once more reflects the importance of good gut health.

As seen in the above example, diet plays an important role—check your diet if breastfeeding or check the ingredients of the formula if bottle-feeding. If your child's eczema is severe, it is recommended that you consult a qualified natural health practitioner or immunologist. In the interim, you can ease the irritation using a water-based cream with evening primrose and calendula oils, adding a few drops of pure essential oils of lavender and German chamomile. Avoid using any petroleum-based skin care or talc on your baby.

Other infections

Fever is the body's way of fighting off an infection. It can be scary when your baby's temperature begins to rise. However, a mild fever is beneficial and should not be suppressed with medications, and it is best to avoid paracetamol or ibuprofen. Homeopathic remedies are safe and very effective for most infant maladies—it is an excellent idea to have a homeopathic first aid kit on hand prior to the birth. An age-old remedy for gently lowering fever in babies is to cut a raw potato in half and place the cut side on the sole of each foot. Pop a sock on to hold the potato in place. Numerous mums have used this remedy—albeit doubting its effectiveness initially—reporting how well it lowered their baby's fever. Once your baby grows a little, you can wipe your baby's legs from the knees down with a cool washcloth and then wrap the legs in a towel. You'll be surprised at how effective this technique is in reducing mild fever—it works on adults too.

Avoiding paracetamol or acetaminophen is recommended, as it needs to be cleared through the liver, and toxicity can result even at low doses. There are also concerns that paracetamol can impede immune responses even when used at the recommended therapeutic doses.[129] In Australia and New Zealand, paracetamol overdose due to medication errors is the leading cause of paediatric acute liver failure.[130]

Rhinitis or sinus congestion is most often linked to dairy, wheat, and sugar consumption, as all increase mucous secretions. Read the ingredients of everything you are feeding your baby to identify possible sources of mucous irritants. If breastfeeding, check your diet for any of these culprits. If congestion persists, there are great homeopathic remedies to ease mucous congestion. Diffusing aniseed essential oil helps to thin mucous so it can easily be cleared via nasal passages. This is also very handy if anyone in the house has a respiratory infection involving nasal congestion.

Avoid exposing your newborn baby to environmental toxins for as long as possible. Remember babies cannot detoxify efficiently so everything they are exposed to—whether it is ingested, applied to skin, or inhaled—needs to be processed.

❖ Skin irritation often reflects gut health.
❖ Avoid all chemicals when it comes to your baby—that includes body care products, fabric softener, tap water.
❖ If breastfeeding, always consider what you are consuming if your baby has any reactions.

18

Baby's emotional Foundations

> It is easier to build strong children than to repair broken adults
> —F. Douglas

How a baby and child respond to stress in their own lives is impacted significantly by the emotional health and stress levels of the mother throughout pregnancy but especially during the first four months of gestation.[131] The impact of stress on brain health begins in the womb. Large human cohort studies have found that prenatal maternal stress affects the brain and behaviour of the offspring, increasing the risk of emotional, cognitive, and behavioural problems later in life.[132] However, it is not only the baby's emotional health that is impacted by the mother's stress—there is also increased risk of preterm delivery and reduced telomere length, possibly accelerating the ageing process of the baby later in life. Iridology assessments on babies reveal distinct signs of stresses that the mother experienced while her baby was still in the uterus. These signs reflect the nervous disposition of that child into adulthood.

Babies feel and mirror the emotions that surround them. If parents are stressed, then the baby will feel this. Some babies respond to stress with unsoothable crying, while others retreat into themselves and remain quiet—even later in life, isolating becomes a coping mechanism. The emotional programming experienced by a baby (from conception onwards) imprints on the amygdala, the part of the brain that processes memory, decision-making, and emotional responses. Have you ever heard someone say they just reacted instinctively? This instinct comes from the amygdala—the brain literally reviews prior life experiences to find how you responded to a similar situation in the past. This is also why it can be difficult to change some behaviours that reside deeply within our psyche, so we should be mindful of this when around babies and children of all ages.

The emotional needs of your baby are just as important as fundamental nutrition. Babies have very few and simple needs once they are born—being fed, having a clean dry bottom, being comfortable, and feeling safe. I once had this explained to me that a baby is born as "love." Every behaviour it witnesses becomes imprinted on its brain as reflecting what "love" means. For example, if the baby cries and you respond by cuddling and soothing it, the baby imprints that "love" means mum or dad holding me, support, care, and safety. On the other hand, if the adults around a crying baby ignore it, then the imprinted message is more like "love means being ignored," a program that may remain with that baby for the rest of its life. I believe we generally underestimate how what we do, feel and how we behave affects our children.

***

❖ Everything your baby experiences creates its blueprint for life.

19

The Baby Blues

> It's OK if you fall apart sometimes. Tacos fall apart and
> we still love them.
> —Unknown

So far, we've been talking about the baby. What about you? How are you feeling? Most new parents agree that sleep deprivation is possibly the biggest challenge during the first few weeks; months; and, in some cases, even years. However, a lot of new mums and dads feel as if they are treading water, just barely coping. Add to this a melancholy mood and a lot of the joy of bringing a new baby home gets buried under emotional highs and lows.

A research team at the University of Tasmania is doing a study looking at antibiotic use during pregnancy and subsequent risk of postnatal depression. There is a growing body of evidence linking antibiotic use with mood disorders resulting from microbiome alterations, and this study is aiming to show whether their use increases the risk of developing postnatal depression. You can follow the progress of this research at https://www.facebook.com/ TheMaternalExperienceStudy/.

Go back to the section on gut health and the importance of your microbiome—just to refresh your memory about how much your gut health affects your entire body, including mental health. This is a timely reminder of why the preparation phase is so important, as is continuing a healthy lifestyle and diet throughout your pregnancy. Taking the right supplements, especially the essential fatty acids, B complex vitamins, and minerals, can significantly help reduce and even prevent, postnatal depression.

In the new mother, a lot of this emotional upheaval can be linked to her hormones rebalancing after the birth. Throughout pregnancy, oestrogen levels continue to rise reaching their peak at forty weeks. Progesterone levels are also much higher than before pregnancy. Add to this the high levels of oxytocin that triggers birth and milk production, as well as feelings of euphoria, the sudden drop in all three hormones after birth will inevitably lead to emotional readjustments. If you know this is coming, you can be prepared for the altered moods.[133] This knowledge will help you not freak out, thinking something is wrong with you—because there is not.

Why do some women experience postnatal depression to the extreme and others none at all or just minimally so? Why does it come to some within a few days after the birth, while others hit rock bottom several weeks later? This can relate back to your genetic SNPs. If you have any alterations in the genes that code for enzymes that help to process hormones, then this can strongly influence your postnatal mental and emotional status. If you have accelerated processing, your body will clear all those hormones very quickly, possibly leaving you feeling suddenly very low. However, if you have SNPs that slow the clearance, you may even remain on a slight "high" for several weeks, experiencing a gradual decline until your body reaches pre-pregnancy levels. It's about knowing your body and being prepared but also understanding why you feel like you do and being reassured there are ways to help you throughout the readjustment phase.

Postnatal depression can affect both parents and ranges from extreme sadness, low energy, anxiety, crying episodes, and irritability to changes in sleeping and eating patterns. The emotions of parents can also affect the baby. All this contributes to overall stress levels, which can snowball out of control. Most new parents admit to being told that having a baby would change their lives, but that they had no idea just how much. Don't let stress and out-of-control emotions ruin this very special time in your and your baby's lives. Take stock of what is important and what is not and begin culling a few time-consuming non-productive activities. Your baby will grow up fast, and while at the beginning it seems like forever, in hindsight, those first few months pass in the blink of an eye.

If you need support, speak to a qualified naturopath, your doctor, or a counsellor to help you through what can be challenging times. There are numerous safe natural remedies that support emotional extremes that are safe to take even while breastfeeding.

***

- ❖ Antibiotics taken during pregnancy have been linked to postnatal depression.
- ❖ Know how your body clears hormones to avoid postnatal depression.
- ❖ Both partners can experience postnatal depression.

20

Stress

> Adopting the right attitude can convert a negative stress into a positive one.
> —Hans Selye

Stress can take on a lot of different shapes and affect people in many different ways. Stress is a biochemical response to a perceived stressor. The stressor—or trigger—can be a thing, event, experience, another person, a thought, or just about anything. Note the use of the word "perceived" because this is part of why some people can breeze through life's turbulence easily, while others can feel stressed or anxious most of the time.

Let me explain the biochemistry of a stress response. Back in the stone age, a stressor would have involved an angry tribesman wielding a club or perhaps a sabre-toothed tiger seeking to make you its next meal. In both instances, the episode would have triggered a response—run or fight for your life. This is known as the fight-flight response or the initial reaction, which is usually brief. During this stage, the adrenal glands release adrenaline and cortisol to help the body respond—fight or run. Energy reserves are mobilised, blood pressure and heart rate increase to better supply nutrients to the muscles, respiration increases so that more oxygen reaches the brain, natural painkillers are released preventatively, and platelets are activated to minimise blood loss in case of injury. Once the danger has passed, our body puts a damper on the inflammatory and immune responses, while promoting the transformation of nutrients, replenishing spent stores of energy (hunger).

These chemical reactions explain how stress can increase blood pressure, cause pain and chronic inflammatory conditions, increase blood sugar levels leading to insulin resistance or diabetes, and cause blood clots when stress is an ongoing state. Moving from the stone age into modern society, the causes of stress have changed significantly yet our body's biochemistry has not. Stress these days takes on a myriad of different forms, each creating the exact same biochemical reactions in the body as did stone age stressors. When these stressful episodes continue repeatedly, our body never gets a chance to rest and repair, resulting in tissue damage and poor health, with chronically elevated cortisol contributing to hormone imbalances, adrenal fatigue, and even autoimmune conditions. Dr Gabor Mate explains how stress can cause illness, even cancer in his book *When the Body Says No*.

Stress affects both male and female fertility but also impacts on the foetus while in the uterus. Research suggests exposure to maternal cortisol and psychosocial stress influences the developing foetus, with consequences for infant stress regulation.[134] This basically means that stress experienced by the mother during pregnancy will affect how that child copes with stressful situations later in life. Let me return to the word "perceived" when it comes to stress and quote Hans Selye once again. "It is not stress that kills us; it is our reaction to it."

I'll share some tools and tips for parents to avoid becoming overly stressed:

- Have realistic expectations of what parenthood will be like.
- Acknowledge that your lives will change and that the baby will become the central focus of all that is for … well, ever, really. It's only the extent of this that changes over time. Initially your new baby is totally reliant on you, twenty-four hours of every single day.
- Remember that you also need to look after yourself—eating well and getting sleep whenever you can.
- You may need to cull some regular activities you both engaged in prior to having a baby. This need not be forever, but it should be realistic.
- Sometimes you just need to ask for help—family, friends, neighbours, professionals. A side note here—I'm one of those people who soldier on and very, very rarely ask for assistance. A friend once gave me a quote. "Ask for help. Receiving is an act of generosity." So, if you need assistance, ask.

The great divide

Roles change once baby comes home. It may be that both parents used to go to work, have a career. Once baby comes into the family, one parent generally remains at home as the primary caregiver. Even though roles are changing, it is still usually the mother who stays at home—at least for a period of time. You may be fortunate enough to have a few weeks together, but eventually dad (or mum) will go back to work. Here is where the great divide can set in.

Consider that mum is at home with the baby all day—more than likely tired after the birth and perhaps struggling with rebalancing hormones and interrupted sleep for feeding. She's trying to keep the household going, preparing meals, and very much looking forward to her partner coming home from work. On the other hand, the partner who has been at work, faced with the daily stressors of the job, is looking forward to coming home for some quiet time. Mum can't wait to have adult conversation, while dad just wants to relax. This scenario may vary depending on your situation, but my point is that the two worlds collide from very different perspectives. Solution—communication! You both need to explain your needs and come to an agreement of how to bridge the chasm. What worked for me? I was at home with the girls for about five years. While the girls were babies, my husband would spend time with them when he got home from work—their special time to help them bond. After all, it is only natural for there to be a stronger bond between mother and baby, who have already had nine months together. This gave him his "winding down" time and me the opportunity to prepare dinner uninterrupted.

Friction resulting from misunderstood needs of your partner is exacerbated if both parents are sleep-deprived. This is just one of the many scenarios that accompany becoming a new parent. Ultimately, you need to look after yourselves and each other, because who else will care for your baby when you fall in a heap?

It's all about perspective

What do I mean by perspective? It is about how you perceive something — your attitude towards it, coupled with beliefs and expectations. This is highly relevant when it relates to having a baby. What are your expectations? What are your fears? With a glut of information on the internet and social media, it can be difficult to navigate through all the advice and recommendations, as well as the newest techniques and experts' advice. If you find suggestions that feel right, save these. Delete those that just do not sit well with you and learn to develop and listen to your own instinct—it is there. In the end, every baby is different with different needs and responses so there is definitely no "one size fits all."

Let's return to your expectations. Some of the fundamentals of having a new baby include its total reliance on you and the fact that its need for food comes first. While some babies settle into a day/night routine within a few weeks, others may take many months. Routines do help a new baby settle faster, so try and keep the daily activities the same. Natalie found that having daily routines for her boys was extremely helpful, for both them and herself. You may find routines stifling—everyone and every family is different.

Many new parents can't wait to show their baby to the world—understandable. This may not be the baby's priority. And going out in the car/bus/train or even aeroplane into busy, noisy, smelly environments can be a significant stress for a newborn. Even shopping centres present an influx of stimuli of many people, voices, music, and general discord. Some cultures keep a new baby in the home for its first three months. If your expectations are to continue being highly social after you have a baby, requiring you to take bubs everywhere you go, consider the impact this may have on your little one. While some babies take outings in their stride, others can become extremely unsettled, reflecting in changed feeding habits or inability to settle and sleep. Particularly during the initial several weeks, until you all find your groove, take your lead from the baby.

Aim to create a calm home—one where there is a feeling of calm, or, in other words, an absence of stress. All too often, a baby's behaviour will be an indicator of stressors, so pay heed to any signs your little one is giving you. We can follow recommendations and guidelines to a tee, but when these just do not work on your baby, you need to be flexible and creative and remain calm. No baby has ever starved itself. But I do question what appears to be a rise in fussy eaters and poor sleepers. The rise in unsettled babies seems to correlate with all the stimulants our modern world provides.

We've already learnt how toxic our world has become and how our children's bodies are receptacles for these from previous generations, but what about all the other stimuli? We live in a world that is wired and Wi-Fi'd to the hilt, with homes often running several "smart" electronic devices, from televisions and vacuum cleaners to refrigerators. Our mobile phones are seldom out of our hands, and a telephone tower is rarely out of sight. Some people live in high-density housing, where the neighbours' use of electronic devices impacts all surrounding residents. I simply can't help but suspect that all these frequencies/waves affect the delicate new and rapidly dividing cells of a baby.

Electronic devices

Stress comes in many and varied forms, including anything that impairs how our body functions. An area most of us do not associate with stress is electromagnetic frequencies, or EMF. These include smartphones, tablets, computers, Wi-Fi, and baby monitors. Jeromy Johnson is an expert in mitigating the negative impacts of EMF exposure.[135] He has a leading website on the topic and consults with individuals, families, and organisations around the world to implement solutions that reduce and eliminate EMF pollution. Jeromy has an advanced degree in civil engineering and has worked in Silicon Valley for fifteen years. After becoming what medical doctors call "electro-hypersensitive" (EHS) in 2011 following extensive exposure to EMF radiation, he embarked on a journey to regain his own health and educate others. You can watch his video, "Wireless Wake-up Call" at https://www.youtube.com/watch?v=F0NEaPTu9oI.

A 2016 meta-study involving EMF revealed that sperm damage was found in twenty-one of twenty-seven studies.[136] Another study in 2017 shows how low-frequency magnetic fields can increase the risk of miscarriage.[137] Children, and especially babies, are more sensitive to their environments and significantly more vulnerable than adults.

For this reason, it is advisable to keep all electronic devices well away from your baby but also away from your abdomen during pregnancy. EMFs can actually penetrate your body's cells and brain, causing varying levels of inflammation and disease. We get so used to using electronic devices we forget they are continually emitting frequencies that affect developing cells (as in a foetus forming inside you). Turn off Wi-Fi and data on your smartphone when not needed and remember to switch off the Wi-Fi modem at home at night and when not in use. These frequencies can influence normal cellular metabolism, including DNA modification.[138]

This can't be stressed enough when it comes to fertility and the health of a rapidly developing foetus and baby.

There are numerous devices touted to help protect from EMF exposure. I've included a few suppliers of these in Appendix 4 that are reasonably priced and appear to work well. But please do your own research to protect yourself and your family.

We live in a modern world where we have all come to rely on electronic devices. Awareness of the dangers can minimise risk to you and your baby. Health impacts of EMF are multiple and varied and can affect any or several of your body's systems, causing a range of symptoms:

- **Neurological** effects may include headaches, dizziness, nausea, difficulty concentrating, memory loss, irritability, depression, anxiety, insomnia, fatigue, weakness, tremors, muscle spasms, numbness, tingling, altered reflexes, muscle and joint paint, or leg/foot pain.
- **Cardiac** symptoms could include palpitations, arrhythmias, pain or pressure in the chest, low or high blood pressure, slow or fast heart rate, or shortness of breath.
- **Respiratory** system impacts include sinusitis, bronchitis, pneumonia, and asthma.
- **Dermatological** symptoms range from skin rash to itching, burning, and facial flushing.
- **Ophthalmologic** impacts may include pain, dryness or burning in the eyes, pressure in or behind the eyes, deteriorating vision, floaters, or cataracts.
- **Other** symptoms may include digestive problems, abdominal pain, enlarged thyroid, or testicular/ovarian pain; dryness of lips, tongue, mouth, or eyes; great thirst or dehydration; nosebleeds or internal bleeding; altered sugar metabolism; immune abnormalities; redistribution of metals within the body; hair loss; pain in the teeth or deteriorating fillings; impaired sense of smell; or ringing in the ears.

Once you begin searching, you'll find a lot of information out there—just beware of those companies only seeking to sell you something. Look for researched articles.[139]

What Are EMFs Anyway?

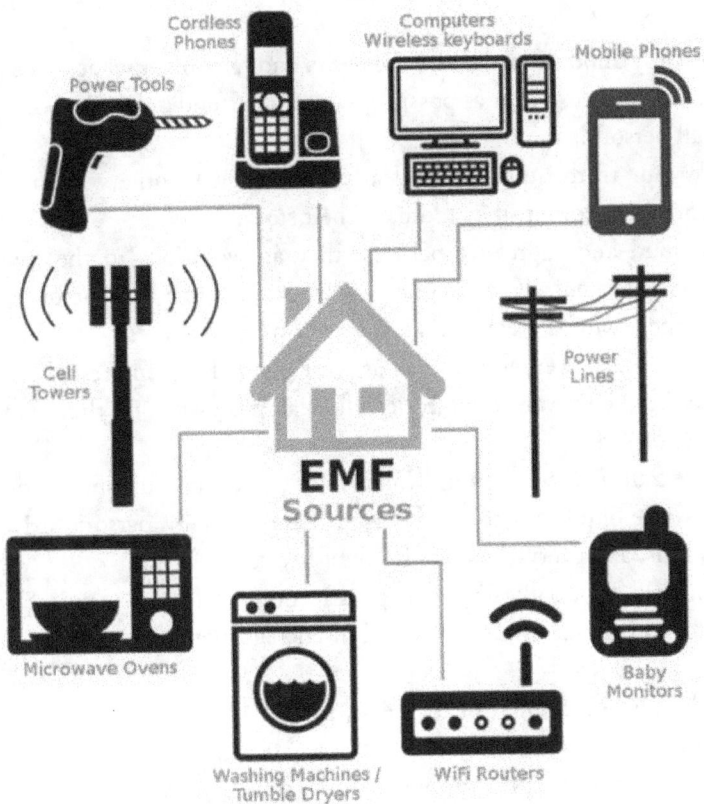

A poem to live by

Desiderata

Go placidly amid the noise and the haste, and remember what peace there may be in silence. As far as possible, without surrender, be on good terms with all persons.

Speak your truth quietly and clearly; and listen to others, even to the dull and the ignorant; they too have their story.

Avoid loud and aggressive persons; they are vexatious to the spirit. If you compare yourself with others, you may become vain or bitter, for always there will be greater and lesser persons than yourself.

Enjoy your achievements as well as your plans. Keep interested in your own career, however humble; it is a real possession in the changing fortunes of time.

Exercise caution in your business affairs, for the world is full of trickery. But let this not blind you to what virtue there is; many persons strive for high ideals, and everywhere life is full of heroism.

Be yourself. Especially do not feign affection. Neither be cynical about love; for in the face of all aridity and disenchantment, it is as perennial as the grass.

Take kindly the counsel of the years, gracefully surrendering the things of youth.

Nurture strength of spirit to shield you in sudden misfortune. But do not distress yourself with dark imaginings. Many fears are born of fatigue and loneliness.

Beyond a wholesome discipline, be gentle with yourself. You are a child of the universe no less than the trees and the stars; you have a right to be here.

And whether or not it is clear to you, no doubt the universe is unfolding as it should. Therefore be at peace with God, whatever you conceive Him to be. And whatever your labors and aspirations, in the noisy confusion of life, keep peace in your soul. With all its sham, drudgery, and broken dreams, it is still a beautiful world. Be cheerful. Strive to be happy.

—Max Ehrmann, early 1920s

❖ Communicate your needs with your partner. And if you need assistance—ask.
❖ Stress is not the problem—it is your reaction to it.
❖ Take care with EMF—the invisible danger.

21

Oxidative Stress

> The main cause of DNA damage is oxidative stress.
> —European Society of Human
> Reproduction and Embryology

What is oxidative stress? It is cell damage caused by free radicals that can be the result of metabolic by-products, external toxins, or lack of nutrients. Oxidative damage was mentioned early in section I, when I explained how free radicals affect sperm quality. Free radicals can affect every single cell in your body. But don't despair—your body has ways of protecting itself, providing you give it what it needs and don't overwhelm it with toxins.

Free radicals are highly reactive and unstable molecules that are made by the body naturally as a by-product of normal metabolism. Free radicals can also be made by the body after exposure to toxins in the environment such as herbicides, pesticides, environmental chemicals, tobacco smoke, and ultraviolet (UV) light. Research carried out by EMR Australia over several years has found another source of oxidative damage. One of the key effects the authors observed was that wireless radiation causes oxidative stress—the generation of free radicals. Oxidative stress is now recognised as an underlying cause of many chronic diseases, such as cardiovascular disease and diabetes, Alzheimer's disease, and depression. Furthermore, health conditions promoted by electromagnetic-induced oxidative stress include allergies and atopic dermatitis, autoimmune diseases such as diabetes, eye conditions, and fertility effects.[140]

Free radicals have a lifespan of only a fraction of a second but, during that time, can damage DNA, sometimes causing mutations that can increase risk of illness or disease. Antioxidants in the foods we eat can neutralise the unstable molecules and reduce the chances of them causing damage. Most antioxidants are found in colourful foods like fruit and vegetables. However, foods provide more than just nutrition and antioxidants—our foods also interact with our genes. Remember the term nutrigenomics mentioned earlier? It is a type of signalling between the foods we eat and our DNA. A much more effective way of preventing oxidative stress and negating free radical damage is to switch on our cells' own defence system—which is exactly the type of communication that happens with nutrigenomics.[141]

Eating a colourful diet high in fruit and vegetables is definitely beneficial for a healthy digestive system and microbiome health. This includes providing the body with adequate levels of protein—particularly methionine, which is a sulfur amino acid and essential for many body processes, including effective detoxification. The brassicas or cruciferous group of vegetables in particular are highly beneficial when it comes to protecting your cells from oxidative damage. Ensuring the body has all the nutrients it needs to quench free radicals is a more sustainable option than trying to make up for a diet high in processed, low-nutrient/high-sugar foods by taking synthetic vitamin C.

22

Post Baby Recovery

Give yourself time.

Many mums who have had one or more children who come into my clinic report feeling tired and run down. During our discussions it often becomes apparent that their health declined following the birth of each child. Rarely do women replenish their nutrient levels following a pregnancy. Many supplement during pregnancy to ensure the health of their unborn child. But what about themselves? Research has now shown that the declining nutrient levels may lead to increased risk of autism in subsequent children —particularly if the pregnancies follow closely. A further consequence of insufficient recovery after a pregnancy can be increased risk of miscarriage. Closely spaced pregnancies were associated with an increase in the odds of a second child being diagnosed with autism, according to a study involving California children. The study, which the *Journal of Paediatrics* published online, showed the sooner conceptions followed the prior birth of a sibling, the greater the likelihood of the second child having an autism diagnosis. The study looked at more than 660,000 second-born children in California between 1992 and 2002. The study measured the time the second child was conceived relative to the first child, and then looked at autism diagnosis of the second sibling. The study found that second children who were conceived less than twelve months after the first child's birth were three times more likely to be diagnosed with autism than children spaced further apart. Second-born children conceived less than two years after the first had almost twice the odds of receiving an autism diagnosis. Unfortunately, the online link to this study has been taken down.

Quite apart from the increase in autism, the mere fact that nutritional deficiencies also increase susceptibility to environmental toxins should motivate all women to ensure their own health is at optimum levels prior to conceiving.[142] Re-read section I of this book about preparing your body for conception and the importance of detoxing well before starting a family, as well as between pregnancies.

Just in case you still can't commit to ensuring your body is nutritionally replete and cleared of most toxins, I'd like you to consider the impacts this may have on your baby. If you are planning on having more children, remember to replenish your body and give it time to recover following the birth of each child.

I'd like to share a little more of Natalie's experience after the traumatic year that followed the birth of her first son. Despite the trauma of her firstborn son's initial year, she decided to have another baby. However, before going down that path, she writes, "I chose to heal myself both physically and mentally until I was over 110 per cent back to my new, normal self."

In addition to replenishing nutrient levels, you need to repair and strengthen your body. Strengthening your pelvic floor and core muscles is important, so seek the guidance of a qualified women's physiotherapist or post-pregnancy personal trainer.

***

- ❖ Give yourself time to fully recover after the birth of your baby
- ❖ Wait until you feel 100% before planning another baby
- ❖ Both parents undertake the pre-conception preparation again

23

Preventative Medicine

> Optimum nutrition is the medicine of tomorrow.
> —Linus Pauling

I'd like to share some of the words Dr Andrew Rostenberg, in his book *Your Genius Body*, uses to explain the concept of the illness continuum—"a trend where each generation is becoming sicker than the one that preceded it".[143] We can attribute this overall decline in health to modern chemical and agricultural practices, as well as our embracing convenience without considering the long-term ramifications. This is why men and women who want to have a child should make every effort to optimise their health *before* getting pregnant.

Preconception and antenatal care may be considered as the ultimate form of preventative medicine. A concept known as "foetal programming" has led to a greater understanding of how a foetus's time in utero can influence its susceptibility to future disease. Foetal exposure to stress, toxins, undernutrition, and obesity has been shown to play a role in the development of many common chronic diseases later in life. The science of epigenetics has uncovered how our body remembers what occurred during our time in the uterus. Epigenetics relates to structural modifications of our genes. Although they don't change our DNA, they do change the way in which our DNA behaves. In this way, epigenetic programming can change characteristics and physical traits of a person during his or her lifetime.

For example, nutrient deficiencies or maternal psychological stress during critical periods of foetal development may not only result in low birth weight and small birth size but may also increase the risk of cardiovascular disease, type 2 diabetes, obesity, and hypertension of that baby later in its life. It has also been found that babies born to mothers who are significantly overweight prior to conception are more likely to develop obesity in adulthood. Other studies have shown that stress during pregnancy may contribute to the child developing neurological disorders, such as impaired cognitive development, behavioural problems, autism, and schizophrenia.

Conclusion

Much of the information I have presented may seem overwhelming, especially if you were largely unaware of all the impacts modern life has on your health. You are not alone in this, as most people I have spoken with in clinic and during the course of writing this book expressed amazement, shock, and surprise at just how toxic our lives have become. This is precisely the reason for writing this book—to enlighten you and share this information so you can feel empowered, rather than overwhelmed. The ultimate form of preventative medicine may lie in improving both parents' health prior to conception.

Will everything in this book guarantee your pregnancy and baby will be perfect? There are no guarantees, especially when it comes to all the things that can influence the millions of cells being created rapidly during the forty weeks of gestation. Unforeseen things can happen, but you can rest assured that, if you have followed the advice herein, you will give your child the very best chance at a healthy start and future life.

If the thought of making changes to your lifestyle and diet seems daunting or "too hard," please consider how hard it is to have a child who is health-challenged. Armed with the information in this book, you now have the power to truly make positive changes to your life and influence the health of the next generations by having a healthy baby.

The foundations of good health and well-being—both yours and your baby's—are good food, clean water, adequate rest and sleep, movement and moderate exercise, and sunshine and fresh air, coupled with avoiding toxic chemicals and damaging frequencies. Prevention is, and always has been, the most successful foundation for good health.

I hope you have enjoyed the journey into how your body works and I wish you and your growing family all the very best for a long and healthy future.

APPENDIX 1

Diet guidelines

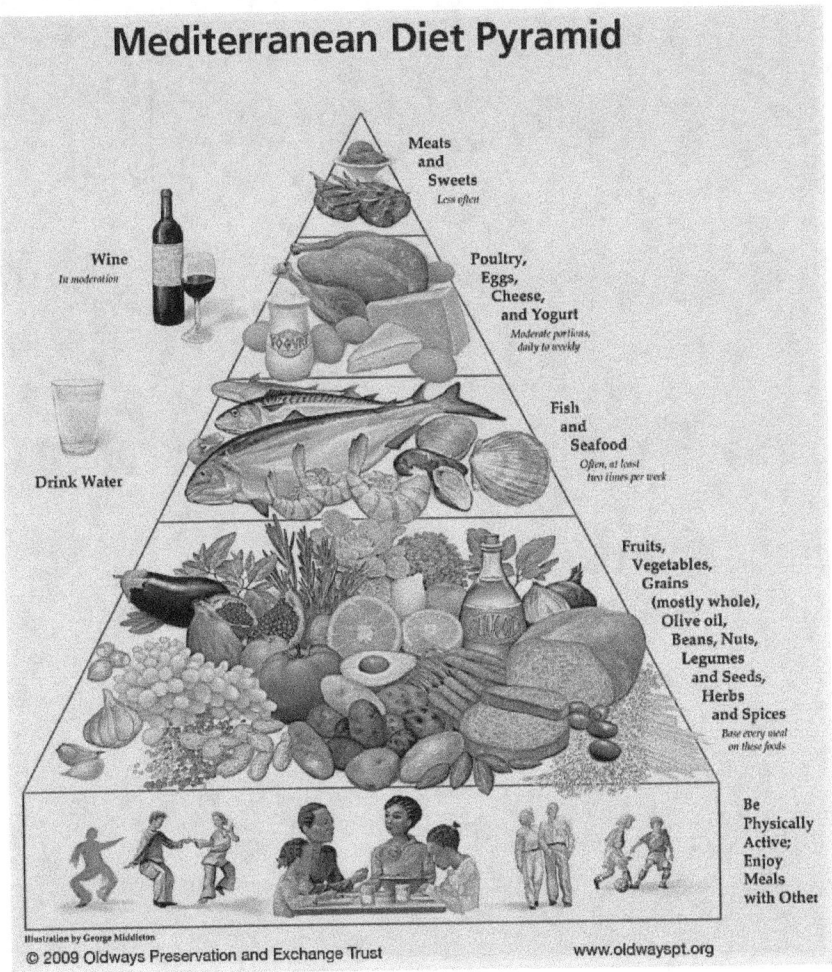

The Mediterranean diet is frequently recommended due to the high plant food content. However, it must also be stressed that, in the Mediterranean regions, most of the products are either home or locally grown. Picked or purchased, freshly harvested foods are then prepared into meals that are mostly shared by several members of the family and/or friends. Time is taken to prepare and eat meals—no comparison to wolfing down a sandwich while sitting at your workplace. While the foods we eat are undeniably important, so too is how we eat them.

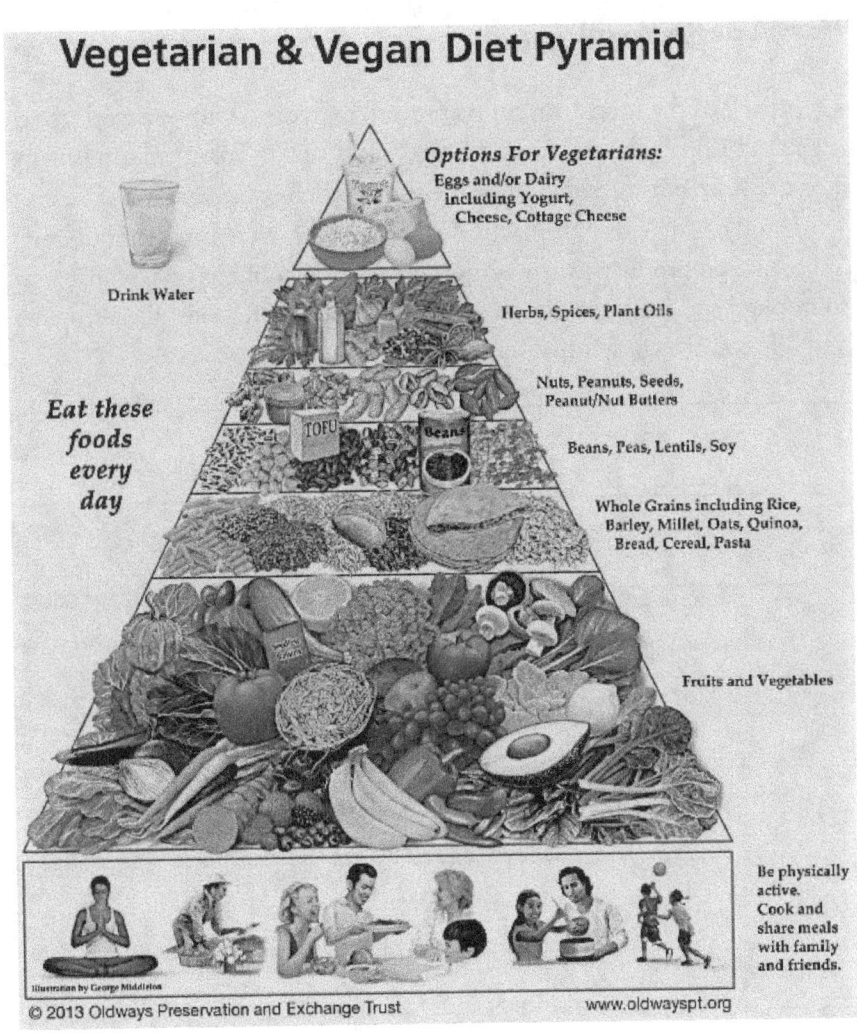

The food pyramids included here are courtesy of Olways Preservation and Exchange Trust. For a wealth of healthy eating information please visit http://www.oldwayspt.org.

How Varied Is Your Diet?

Keep track of the foods you eat (yes, every ingredient) for one week to see if you can fill fifty boxes! A varied diet that is rich in colourful foods helps feed a diverse gut microbiome and ensures a rich spectrum of nutrients.

Handy hint—red and white onions count as two different foods. Wheat-based products, such as bread and pasta, count as one, whilst a rye sourdough and spelt sourdough count as two different foods. Herbs, spices, and oils count as individual ingredients.

What's on Your Plate?

The ideal balance of nutrients is received when your plate is made up of a quarter protein, a quarter starches or carbohydrates, and a half vegetables. The image here is one I created and have used extensively in clinic to assist patients when it comes to portion sizes and meal composition.

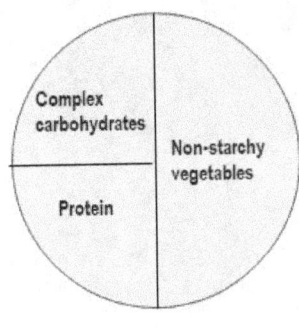

Portion Sizes:

Cup your hands together, side by side palms upward. This will give you an indication of how big your portion sizes should be.

Breakfast: 80% surface area of both your palms

Snacks: 80% of the surface area of one palm

Lunch & Dinner: 100% surface area of both your palms

Protein should be size and thickness of one palm. During pregnancy or higher protein needs, increase to first crease of fingers.

Every person's body is different with varying needs for nutrients. We all have the perfect measures with us at all times—our hands.

APPENDIX 2

Nutrition Guidelines

Preconception and Pregnancy Nutrition

Before starting a family, it is important to consider nutritional preparation for both the prospective mother and prospective father. Proper preconception nutrition may assist in falling pregnant, help maintain a viable pregnancy, and produce a healthy baby.

What follows is a list of preconception and pregnancy guides for the prospective mother and a preconception guide for the prospective father.

Nutrition for the Mum-to-Be

Nutrient	Why it is needed and food sources
Protein	Protein is vital for the number and quality of eggs (ova) produced, the fertilisation process, and early development of the embryo. It's also essential for baby's brain development and function. Essential amino acids are required to prevent mutations. Eat high-quality animal protein (lean meat, poultry, fish), yoghurt, seeds, nuts, sprouted grains, and organic free-range eggs. If your diet is vegan, protein combining is vital to receive adequate amounts. See sources below. Avoid smoked fish or meat products, including bacon. Upon conception, increase intake by 10 to 30 per cent of good quality protein.
Vitamin A	Lack of vitamin A may hinder conception or lead to miscarriage or, in full-term pregnancy, may result in birth defects (cleft palates). Best source is beta-carotene. Food sources—apricots, butter, egg yolk, fish liver oils; red, orange, dark green, and yellow vegetables (red capsicum, spinach, carrots, sweet potatoes); orange fruits (papaya, tomatoes)

Nutrient	Why it is needed and food sources
Vitamin B complex	The B vitamins are important to keep the hormonal balance, which is essential for the early development of the embryo and the smooth progression of the pregnancy. The B complex is essential for methylation. Cooking and processing can result in between 40 and 70 per cent loss of nutrients.
Thiamine (B1)	Thiamine is essential for maintaining pregnancy and preventing abnormalities. Food sources—asparagus, beef, brewer's yeast, lamb, legumes, liver, rye, spirulina, whole grains, nuts, seeds, wheat germ
Riboflavin (B2)	Insufficient amounts of riboflavin in the diet may lead to infertility or malformation of the embryo. Food sources—almonds, asparagus, avocados, barley grass, beans, currants, eggs, whole milk and dairy products, mushrooms, spinach, whole grains, broad beans, organ meats, sprouts
Niacin (B3)	Essential for energy production in every cell, niacin is a cofactor for enzymes; it aids synthesis of fatty acids—helps prevent DNA damage. Food sources—almonds, beef, chicken, eggs, fish, legumes, peanuts, salmon, sardines, sunflower seeds, yeast
Pantothenic acid (B5)	Pantothenic acid helps build body cells and supports normal growth and development of the central nervous system. Readily available in most foods including avocado, baker's yeast, beans, sunflower seeds, mushrooms, plain yoghurt, squash, peanuts, green vegetables, broccoli, baked potato, legumes, cooked egg yolk, lentils, liver, oranges, peas, sweet potatoes, whole grains
Pyridoxine (B6)	Pyridoxine increases chances of conception. Food sources—animal protein foods, spinach, potatoes, bananas, salmon, sunflower seeds

Nutrient	Why it is needed and food sources
Folic acid (B9)	Folic acid is the most important of the B complex to be taken pre-conceptually, as it is needed in the very early stages of pregnancy for the formation of organs. Note: It's important to replenish supplies of folic acid when coming off the Pill or other hormone contraception. Food sources—barley, beans, eggs, endive, green leafy vegetables, asparagus, spinach, lentils, black-eyed peas, Romaine lettuce, broccoli, sunflower seeds, cooked beets, sprouts, organic soybeans
Cobalamin (B12)	Cobalamin enhances fertility; a deficiency may cause spinal cord damage in the infant. Note that vegetarians should beware, as the main source of cobalamin is animal products. Food sources—meat, fish, dairy, eggs
Choline	Choline supports methylation, aids development of nerve tissues, aids cell membrane structure, and supports memory and brain development in foetus. Food sources—beans, beef and chicken liver, egg yolk, lecithin, lentils, whole milk, peanuts, split peas, organic soybeans, spinach, whole grains
Vitamin C	Vitamin C assists with ovulation, heavy bleeding, and infertility and is necessary for a continuing pregnancy. If using supplements, ensure they contain bioflavonoids (rutin, hesperidin, quercetin, and Vitamin E) to assist with absorption. Food sources—parsley, strawberries, broccoli, green vegetables, aloe vera juice, blackcurrants, Brussels sprouts, guava, pawpaw, citrus fruits capsicum, pineapple, raw cabbage, sweet potatoes
Vitamin D	Vitamin D is essential for growth of bones and teeth, as well as calcium and phosphorus absorption. A deficiency is a factor in deformities. Sources—sunshine (converted to vitamin D by our body); milk, fish oils, oily fish, egg yolk, sprouted seeds, butter

Nutrient	Why it is needed and food sources
Vitamin E	Known as the "fertility vitamin," vitamin E ensures conception and a healthy pregnancy and facilitates easy delivery. Food sources—almonds, apricot oil, beef, corn, egg yolk, hazelnuts, wheatgerm, plant oils
Essential fatty acids	Required for the development of the child's brain, nervous system, walls of all cells, and the baby's body functions, essential fatty acids can also protect against cot death. Food sources—flax seed oil, fish oils, sesame seed oil, spirulina, organic soybeans, lecithin, mackerel, sardines, tuna, salmon, seaweed, tofu
Calcium	Essential for the development of baby's bones and teeth and uterine muscle tone, calcium also assists with conception. Food sources—sardines, molasses, vegetables (peas, beans, broccoli, cauliflower), almonds, egg yolk, organic soybeans, turnips, cucumber (skin on), whole milk, dairy products
Zinc	Zinc improves reproductive tone, normal egg production, brain development, and DNA. Food sources—meat, fish, seeds, wheat germ, onions, maple syrup, mushrooms, whole grains, nuts, peas, carrots, herrings, oysters, tomatoes, capsicum, egg yolk, ginger
Magnesium	Magnesium is important for muscle tone and hormonal balance. Deficiency may lead to retarded foetal development, miscarriage, or low birth weight. It's essential to avoid toxaemia in later pregnancy. Food sources—whole grains, green vegetables, nuts, cod, lima beans, figs, molasses, parsnips, soybeans, kelp, eggs
Manganese	Manganese is essential for a viable pregnancy, as well as for bone, heart, and nervous system. Food sources—leafy green vegetables, peas, beans, whole grains, nuts, almonds, avocado, buckwheat, coconuts, corn, kelp, liver, olives, pecans, pineapple juice, walnuts, turnips, carrots, broccoli, legumes

Nutrient	Why it is needed and food sources
Iodine	Iodine is essential for both thyroid function and hormone balance. Deficiency may lead to cretinism. It's important to note that, like copper and iron, iodine is dangerous in excess (pregnancy needs 170 mg/day). Food sources—Celtic sea salt, plain yoghurt, buttermilk, eggs, garlic, asparagus, mushrooms, oysters
Iron	Essential for the baby's bloodstream, brain, bone, and eye development, as well as rate of growth, iron is also important for general fertility. Note, *if using a supplement, do not use ferrous oxide or ferrous sulphate; take supplements on alternate days away from coffee/tea and milk.* Food sources—meat, organ meats (liver, kidney), eggs, leafy green vegetables, almonds, avocado, parsley, pine nuts, soybeans, wheat germ, yeast
Copper	Copper in excess can cause infertility with deficiency linked to foetal resorption. Most urban dwellers have sufficient (or too much). If in doubt, do an HTMA. Food sources—avocado, broccoli, buckwheat, legumes, whole rice, liver, cauliflower, chocolate, kale, molasses, mushrooms, green peas and beans, peanuts, walnuts, oysters, soybeans, wheat germ, bran, seeds, oysters, perch, prunes
Trace minerals	Trace minerals include boron, selenium (antioxidant), chromium (blood sugar), potassium (blood pressure), phosphorous (bone growth), and silicon (bone and connective tissue). Deficiencies have been linked with cot death and Down's syndrome. Food sources—whole foods
CoQ10	CoQ10 is a fat-soluble compound that your body makes naturally and stores in the mitochondria of your cells, particularly in vital organs like the heart, lungs, and liver. It creates energy within your cells and functions as an antioxidant, protecting your cells from free radical damage that can lead to serious diseases. Food sources—organ meats; fatty fish; organic soy products, and vegetables, especially broccoli, nuts, and seeds Nutrients that support the body's own manufacture of CoQ10 include tyrosine; folate; and vitamins C and B2, B3, B5, B6, and B12.

If seeking to supplement, please consult a qualified naturopath for quality products and personalised assessment of need.

Avoid megavitamins because

- high levels of folic acid can mask a B12 deficiency,
- too much B6 can be toxic and lead to numbness in hands and feet,
- too much copper can decrease zinc levels and fertility,
- too much Vitamin A is toxic, and
- too much iron affects zinc absorption.

The adage of "if a little is good, more is better" does *not* apply.

Avoid alcohol, caffeine, refined carbohydrates, saturated fats, chemicals and additives, processed (delicatessen) meats, green potatoes (contain mutagenic substances), soft drinks, and energy drinks.

Limit processed foods. Energy should be in the form of complex carbohydrates—vegetables and good grains like brown rice, organic oats, millet, barley, rye, spelt, and quinoa.

Limit processed salt, sugar, and dairy products. Use authentic Himalayan rock salt on food to maintain electrolytes.

Eat lots of fresh fruit and vegetables, whole organic grains, and plenty of protein.

Regular exercise—our bodies are made to move.

Rest is essential—quality sleep is invaluable.

Nutrition for the Dad-to-Be

Nutrient	Why it's needed and food sources
Protein	Protein is vital for optimum functioning of the testes, sperm production and viability, and the fertilisation process. Food sources—high-quality animal protein (lean meat, fish), yoghurt, seeds, nuts, sprouted grains, and free-range eggs Avoid smoked fish or meat products, including bacon.
Zinc	Vital for viable sperm count, motility, and a high percentage of live sperm in the semen, zinc is the *most important* mineral for male reproductive health. Take daily for at least six, preferably twelve months before conception. Test for dose needed. Food sources—meat, fish, seeds, wheat germ, onions, maple syrup, mushrooms, whole grains, nuts, peas, carrots, herring, oysters, tomatoes, capsicum, egg yolk, ginger, herrings
Manganese	Deficiency of manganese can lead to a total lack of sperm. Food sources—leafy vegetables, peas, beans, whole grains, nuts, almonds, avocado, buckwheat, coconuts, corn, kelp, liver, olives, organ meats, pecans, pineapple juice, turnips, carrots, broccoli, legumes
Potassium	Potassium deficiency can reduce sperm motility. Food sources—all vegetables, whole grains, apricots, avocado, banana, citrus fruit, dates, herring, parsley, potato, sardines
Magnesium	Magnesium is important for healthy sperm. Food sources—whole grains, green vegetables, nuts, cod, lima beans, figs, molasses, parsnips, soybeans, kelp, eggs
Calcium	Calcium is essential to trigger proper cell division following fertilisation of the ovum. Food sources—sardines, molasses, peas, beans, broccoli, cauliflower, almonds, egg yolk, organic soybeans, turnips, cucumber (skin on) whole milk, dairy products

Nutrient	Why it's needed and food sources
Chromium	Chromium is important blood sugar regulation. Food sources—brewer's yeast, mushrooms, black pepper, liver, beef, whole grains, beets, apples, egg yolk, molasses, nus, oysters, peanuts, potato, prunes
Selenium	Deficiency of selenium decreases sperm production and mortality and can lead to deformities (including Down's syndrome). It is lost through frequent ejaculation. Food sources—alfalfa, barley, broccoli, Brazil nuts, tuna, herring, bran, brewer's yeast, wheat germ, eggs, onions, garlic, liver, cabbage, tomatoes, celery, mackerel, oysters, peanuts, onions, turnips
Essential fatty acids	Deficiency of essential fatty acids can lead to general impairment of testicular function and even chromosome defects. Males need more than females. Food sources—fish oils, sesame seed oil, spirulina, organic soybeans, lecithin, mackerel, sardines, tuna, salmon, seaweed, tofu
Vitamin A	Vitamin A is needed for sperm production, healthy testes, and conversion of cholesterol to testosterone. Food sources—apricots, butter, egg yolk, fish liver oils; red, orange, dark green, and yellow vegetables (red capsicum, spinach, sweet potatoes, carrots); orange fruits (papaya, tomatoes)
Vitamin B complex	The particular B vitamins needed are B5 for healthy testes and B12 to increase sperm count and motility. All B vitamins are useful and will help counteract stress reactions. Always take a balanced B vitamin formula if supplementing.
Vitamin C	Necessary to prevent sperm clumping, which causes infertility, vitamin C, when levels are good, can protect against genetic abnormalities and increase sperm motility. Take with bioflavonoids. Food sources—parsley, strawberries, broccoli, green vegetables, aloe vera juice, blackcurrants, Brussels sprouts, guava, pawpaw, citrus fruits, capsicum, pineapple, raw cabbage, sweet potatoes

Nutrient	Why it's needed and food sources
Vitamin E	Vitamin E is required for good sperm count. Deficiency can lead to total lack of sperm. Food sources—almonds, apricot oil, beef, corn, egg yolk, hazelnuts, wheat germ, plant oils
Protein	Protein is necessary for the optimum functioning of testes and a good source of amino acids. Deficiency can lead to chromosome aberrations. Food sources—high-quality animal protein (lean meat, fish); yoghurt; seeds, nuts, and sprouted gains; and organic free-range eggs Note, if vegan, protein combining is vital to receive adequate amounts.
CoQ10	CoQ10 is a fat-soluble compound that your body makes naturally and stores in the mitochondria of your cells, particularly in vital organs like the heart, lungs, liver, and sperm. It creates energy for sperm motility and within your cells and functions as an antioxidant, protecting your cells from free radical damage that can lead to serious diseases. Food sources—organ meats; fatty fish; organic soy products; and vegetables, especially broccoli, nuts, and seeds Nutrients that support the body's own manufacture of CoQ10 include tyrosine; folate; and vitamins C and B2, B3, B5, B6, and B12.

Eat lots of fresh fruit, vegetables, and whole grains.

Reduce intake of refined carbohydrates, animal fats, processed salt, sugar, and dairy products.

Don't smoke. Nicotine can lead to atrophy of the testicles, low sperm count, poor motility, and deformities.

Little or no alcohol should be consumed (perhaps an occasional standard glass of wine or beer).

Avoid coffee, chemicals, additives, non-essential medication, drugs, artificial sweeteners, soft drinks, and energy drinks.

Regular exercise is a must.

Note that heat and pressure kill sperm. Avoid hot baths.

Essential Fatty Acids

Essential Fatty Acid	Omega-3	Omega-6	Omega-9
Mono or poly	Polyunsaturated Linolenic acid	Polyunsaturated Linoleic acid	Monounsaturated
Made by	Essential—can't be synthesised by the human body	Essential—can't be synthesised by the human body	The human body can make omega-9
Benefits	✓ Cell membranes ✓ Mental health ✓ Heart health ✓ Decreases liver fat ✓ Healthy weight management ✓ Reduces inflammation ✓ Infant brain development ✓ Bone health ✓ Circulation ✓ Lowers cholesterol ✓ Skin, kidney and liver health ✓ Sperm motility and concentration	✓ Reduces nerve pain ✓ Bone health ✓ Decreases blood pressure ✓ Lower risk of heart disease ✓ Reduces ADHD symptoms ✓ May alleviate rheumatoid arthritis symptoms	✓ Reduces cardiovascular risk

Essential Fatty Acid	Omega-3	Omega-6	Omega-9
Sources	Oily cold-water fish, including sardines, salmon, mackerel, herrings, ocean trout, tuna; green leafy vegetables like kale, spinach; chia seeds, flaxseed oil, blackcurrant seed oil	Olive oil, walnut, evening primrose oil, borage oil, and most vegetables contain low levels	Almond oil, peanut oil, avocado oil, olive oil
Requires zinc, B6, insulin, and magnesium	EPA and DHA	GLA and CLA	Oleic acid—major fatty acid in human milk and nerve membranes

Protein Content Guide

FOOD SOURCES AND QUANTITIES OF PROTEIN

Meats
Beef steak, grilled (130g)	34.5g
Mince, cooked (130g)	30g
Liver (beef), grilled (85g raw)	23g
Lamb chop, grilled (95g raw)	11g
Pork, cooked (100g raw)	23g
Ham, 2 slices (50g)	5.5g

Chicken
White/dark meat (100g raw)	28g
Breast (80g raw)	22g
¼ chicken, roasted (100g)	25g

Fish
White fish (100g raw)	17.5g
Canned fish	
Tuna (50g)	15g
Salmon (50g)	10g
Sardines (35g)	9g
Shellfish	
Crabmeat (100g)	20g
Prawns (50g)	12g
Oysters, raw (6 medium)	6.5g
Crayfish/lobster (whole)	22g

Eggs
1 large, whole	6g
Egg yolk	3g
Egg white	3g

Grains
Wheat (100g)	9.4g
Oats (100g)	11g
Millet (100g)	9.6g
Quinoa (100g)	14g
Wholemeal bread, 2 slices	6g
Pasta, ½ cup	8g

Rice
White, cooked (½ cup)	2g
Brown, cooked (½ cup)	2.5g

Nuts & Seeds
Almonds (30g)	6g
Almond butter (1 Tbsp)	2.43g
Cashews (30g)	5g
Peanut butter (1 Tbsp)	7.5g
Walnuts (12-20 halves)	7g
Sesame seeds (1 Tbsp)	2.5g
Sunflower seeds (30g)	6.5g
Tahini (1 Tbsp)	3.5g

Fruit
Avocado (½ medium)	2.5g
Figs, dried (3)	2g
Dates (4–5)	0.7g

FOOD SOURCES AND QUANTITIES OF PROTEIN

Milk/dairy		Vegetables	
Full cream (250ml)	8.5g	Beans, kidney, cooked (½ cup)	7g
Skim 250ml	9g	Baked beans (½ cup)	7g
Soy milk (250ml)	5-10g	Chickpeas (½ cup)	6g
Yogurt (200g)	8g	Beans, soy, cooked (½ cup)	11g
Cheese, firm (30g)	7.5g	Tofu, firm (150g raw)	10g
Reduced fat (30g)	25g	Mung bean sprouts (½ cup)	1.5g
Cottage cheese (30g)	5g	Bean sprouts (½ cup)	8g
Ricotta (30g)	3.3g	Lentils, cooked (½ cup)	9g
Feta (30g)	4g	Mixed vegies (100g)	1.4g
		Broccoli (1 cup)	2.7g

Daily protein needs calculation

- Your ideal body weight ____ kg x 0.8 = ____ grams of protein needed daily
- For vegetarians, multiply by 1.0, and vegans, by 1.2

Fibre Content of Common Foods

For maximum fibre, consume foods with skin on but ensure the food is organic or at least unsprayed.

Common foods that provide fibre	
Grains 10 grams	1 cup of rolled oats, raw 2 cups of barley, cooked 2 cups cooked quinoa 2 cobs of sweet corn (organic) 3 slices of organic whole rye bread 5 slices of wholemeal bread ¾ cup of natural bran 3½ cups cooked brown rice 8 cups cooked white rice
Legumes 15 grams	1 cup mixed beans 1 cup cooked peas 1 cup baked beans 1¼ cup cooked lentils 1 cup cooked chickpeas 8 grams of tofu
Nuts and seeds 5 grams	90 grams almonds 1 cup peanuts 100 grams pistachio nuts ¾ cup pecans ¾ cup sunflower seeds
Vegetables 10 grams	3 cups steamed mixed vegetables 3 cups carrots 2 cups cabbage 3 cups beetroot 3 cups cooked broccoli 1 cup steamed spinach 2 cups cooked sweet potato 2–3 medium steamed potatoes with skin

Common foods that provide fibre	
Fruit **5 grams**	2 medium apples, skin on 3 oranges 100 grams dried figs 10 dried apricots (organic, unsprayed, sulfur-free) 2–3 bananas 2 passionfruit 400 grams blueberries 4 kiwi fruit peeled 6–7 nectarines 1 medium pear, skin on 20 grams prunes 2 ½ cups organic strawberries ½ avocado

Aim to eat between 30 and 50 grams of fibre every day.

Essential Amino Acids

There are nine essential amino acids, each of which performs a number of important jobs in your body[144]:

1. **Phenylalanine.** Your body turns this amino acid into the neurotransmitters tyrosine, dopamine, epinephrine, and norepinephrine. It plays an integral role in the structure and function of proteins and enzymes and the production of other amino acids.
2. **Valine.** This is one of three branched-chain amino acids (BCAAs) on this list. That means it has a chain branching off from one side of its molecular structure. Valine helps stimulate muscle growth and regeneration and is involved in energy production.
3. **Threonine.** This is a principal part of structural proteins, such as collagen and elastin, which are important components of your skin and connective tissue. It also plays a role in fat metabolism and immune function.
4. **Tryptophan.** Often associated with drowsiness, tryptophan is a precursor to serotonin, a neurotransmitter that regulates your appetite, sleep, and mood.
5. **Methionine.** This amino acid plays an important role in metabolism and detoxification. It's also necessary for tissue growth and the absorption of zinc and selenium, minerals that are vital to your health.
6. **Leucine.** Like valine, leucine is a BCAA that is critical for protein synthesis and muscle repair. It also helps regulate blood sugar levels, stimulates wound healing, and produces growth hormones.
7. **Isoleucine.** The last of the three BCAAs, isoleucine is involved in muscle metabolism and is heavily concentrated in muscle tissue. It's also important for immune function, haemoglobin production, and energy regulation
8. **Lysine.** Lysine plays major roles in protein synthesis, calcium absorption, and the production of hormones and enzymes. It's also important for energy production, immune function, and the production of collagen and elastin.

9. **Histidine.** Your body uses this amino acid to produce histamine, a neurotransmitter vital to immune response, digestion, sexual function, and sleep-wake cycles. It's critical for maintaining the myelin sheath, a protective barrier that surrounds your nerve cells.

As you can see, essential amino acids are at the core of many vital processes

Nutrient sources and actions courtesy of Henry Osiecki.[145]

APPENDIX 3

Labs and Tests Guide

Blood Pathology

Preconception assessment of blood parameters (and urine where applicable) is highly recommended. Some tests are the same for men and women. Specific tests have been identified accordingly below. Ask your doctor for these tests.

Both men and women

- ☑ Serum chemistry—E/LFT, eGFR (includes kidney and liver function, electrolyte levels, pH)
- ☑ Full blood count (red/white blood information and immune status)
- ☑ CRP (inflammation marker)
- ☑ ESR (inflammation and blood viscosity marker)
- ☑ Iron studies (free and stored iron levels)
- ☑ HbA1c (early indicator of insulin resistance)
- ☑ Plasma zinc
- ☑ Serum copper + caeruloplasm
- ☑ Vitamin D
- ☑ Red blood cell selenium
- ☑ Homocysteine (inflammation marker, indicator of B vitamin metabolism, pre-eclampsia, miscarriage, NTDs)
- ☑ HDL/LDL/Trig (cholesterol)
- ☑ Infective screen—EBV, CMV, HSV-1/2, HHV, mycoplasma, ureaplasma[1]
- ☑ Full STI
- ☑ Blood group
- ☑ SAM, SAH, SAM:SAH (indicator of methylation capacity)

---

[1] Any residual viral infection can be passed on to the foetus so needs to be cleared prior to conception.

Women only

- TSH
- fT4
- fT3
- rT3 (all the above relate to thyroid function)
- TPO & Tg and TRAbs (thyroid antibodies)
- Urinary creatinine
- Urinary iodine
- Hormone panel to include FSH, LH, E2, prolactin, DHEA-S, testosterone, FAI, SHBG, AMH, 17-OHP4

Men only

- Testosterone—free and bound, oestrogen, prolactin, FSH, LH, DHEAs, SHBG
- PSA—depending on age
- TSH

Semen analysis - https://www.clinicallabs.com.au/patient/semen-analysis-collection-centre-locations/

Hair Tissue Mineral Analysis

InterClinical Laboratories	https://interclinical.com.au/htma-pathology/
	Phone (02) 9693 2888
	6/10 Bradford St, Alexandria, 2015 NSW Australia
Doctors Data	https://www.doctorsdata.com/Hair-Elements
	Phone US & Canada 800 323 2784
	Phone Global +1 630 377 8139
	3755 Illinois Avenue, St. Charles, IL 60174-2420 USA

Functional Pathology	Laboratory
Organic acid test	Mosaic Diagnostics
Urinary toxins	Mosaic Diagnostics
Mould and food allergies	Mosaic Diagnostics
Chemical toxins	Mosaic Diagnostics
	https://mosaicdx.com/
	Phone toll free US 800-288-0383
	8400 W 110th Street, Overland Park, KS 66210 U.S.A.
Hormones/neurotransmitters	Doctors Data—HuMAP
Stool analysis	Doctors Data—GI360
Urinary toxins	Doctors Data
Drinking water analysis	Doctors Data
Methylation profile	Doctors Data
Hormones	Doctors Data
	Phone US & Canada 800 323 2784
	Phone Global +1 630 377 8139
	3755 Illinois Avenue, St. Charles, IL 60174-2420 USA
Hormones	Precision Analytical—DUTCH
	https://dutchtest.com/
	Phone +1 (503) 687-2050
	3138 NE Rivergate Street, Suite #301C McMinnville, OR 97128 USA
DNA	DNA-Life
	https://www.dnalife.healthcare/products/dna

APPENDIX 4

Suppliers

I declare that I do not have a vested interest in any of the companies mentioned in this appendix. Nor do I receive any financial or incentive benefits from any of them. I recommend these companies due to the quality of their products and services.

Water filters
Which filter?

www.biopure.com
https://www.foodmatters.com/article/what-water-filter-should-I-be-using

Frequency therapy

www.ryfemax.com.au

EMF device protection

Orgone Effects Australia
Shop: 23/50 Guelph Street Somerville, Vic. 3912 (by appointment only)
Tel: +613 5977 7162
https://orgoneffectsaustralia.com.au/

Life Energy Solutions
27 Cherub Place, West Harbour,
Auckland 0618 New Zealand
Tel: +649 416 6959
https://lifeenergysolutions.com/

Don Morrison
https://donamorrison.com/

Quality essential oils

http://essentialtherapeutics.com.au/
https://seoc.com.au/

International brands and suppliers

Fish Oils	**Nordic Naturals** https://www.nordic.com/
United Kingdom and Europe	**Your Health Basket** https://yourhealthbasket.co.uk/ **Mannayan GmbH & Co.KG** Unterer Anger 15 80331 Munich Germany www.mannayan.com
Homeopathic prophylaxis	**Dr Isaac Golden and Anita Di Stasio** PO Box 695, Gisborne, 3437 Vic Australia Clinic phone: +613 5427 0880 Email: homstudy@bigpond.com www.homstudy.net or consult your local classical homeopath

APPENDIX 5

Recommended Reading

Title	Author	ISBN
Your Genius Body: A Guide for Optimizing Your Genes & Changing Your Life	Andrew Rostenberg, DC	978-0-578-39326-1
Toxic Legacy: How the Weedkiller Glyphosate Is Destroying Our Health and the Environment	Stephanie Seneff, PhD	978-1-60358-929-1
Eat Like the Animals: What Nature Teaches Us about the Science of Healthy Eating	David Raubenheimer and Stephen J. Simpson	978-1-4607-5869-4
The Nutrient Bible, 9th edition	Henry Osiecki	978-1-8752-3954-2
Toxic Bite: An Investigation into Truth Decay	Bill Kellner-Read	1-904015-00-X
Trace Elements and Other Essential Nutrients: Clinical Application of Tissue Mineral Analysis	David L. Watts, DC, PhD	1-885676-24-7
The Rain Barrel Effect	Dr Stephen Cabral	978-1-9757-7483-7
Dr Libby's Real Food Kitchen	Dr Libby Weaver	978-0-473-29900-2

Title	Author	ISBN
James Duigan's Blueprint for Health	James Duigan	978-1-911216-64-3
A Balanced Approach to PCOS	Melissa Groves Azzaro	978-1-628604-13-9

There are many great resources available, and this list represents just a few to get you started.

GLOSSARY

Term	Meaning
ADD, ADHD.	Attention deficit disorder, attention deficit hyperactivity disorder.
amygdala.	One of two almond-shaped clusters of nuclei located deep and medially within the temporal lobes of the brain's cerebrum in complex vertebrates, including humans. Shown to perform a primary role in the processing of memory, decision-making, and emotional responses, the amygdalae are considered part of the limbic system.
analgesic.	Pain relief medication.
anticoagulant.	Anti-clotting medication.
anti-sperm antibodies.	Like the name says, anti-sperm antibodies fight sperm. It happens when the immune system mistakenly targets sperm in a man's semen as an invader and damages or kills it. Anti-sperm antibodies aren't common. Both men and women can make them.
atopy.	A disorder marked by the tendency to develop localised immediate hypersensitivity reactions to allergens such as pollen, food, and so on and is manifested by hay fever, asthma, eczema, or similar allergic conditions. Atopy is generally considered to be caused by the interaction of environmental and genetic factors.
blastocyst.	A structure formed in the early embryonic development of mammals. In humans, blastocyst formation begins about five days after fertilisation. About seven days after fertilisation, the blastocyst undergoes implantation, embedding into the endometrium of the uterine wall.
BPA.	Bisphenol A, a chemical compound primarily used in the manufacturing of various plastics. BPA is a xenoestrogen, exhibiting hormone-like properties that mimic the effects of oestrogen in the body.
brassica vegetables.	A group of vegetables also known as cruciferous vegetables that includes broccoli, Brussels sprouts, cauliflower, cabbage, bok choy, choy sum, kohlrabi, rutabaga, turnip, mustard greens, collard greens, and kale.

Term	Meaning
cerebral cortex.	Also called grey matter, your brain's outermost layer of nerve cell tissue. Your cerebral cortex plays a key role in memory, thinking, learning, reasoning, problem-solving, emotions, consciousness and functions related to your senses.
CLA.	Conjugated linoleic acid found mostly in the meat and dairy products derived from ruminants.
cleft palate.	An abnormal condition in which the two plates of the skull that form the hard palate (roof of the mouth) are not completely joined, resulting from incomplete fusion during embryonic development. Cleft palate may involve only the uvula or extend through the entire palate.
club-foot.	Deformity of the foot, usually marked by a curled shape or twisted position of the ankle, heel, and toes.
CMV.	Cytomegalovirus, a member of the herpes family associated with pneumonia
CNS.	Central nervous system, consisting of the brain and spinal cord.
congenital.	Relating to a condition that is present at birth, as a result of either heredity or environmental influences.
dioxin.	Any of several carcinogenic, mutagenic, and teratogenic polychlorinated heterocyclic aromatic hydrocarbons that can occur as impurities in petroleum-derived herbicides and as by-products of manufacturing chemicals and burning fuels and waste. Any of a broad range of toxic or carcinogenic halogenated polycyclic compounds that occur as by-products of herbicides.
DNA fragmentation.	The separation or breaking of DNA strands into pieces.
E. coli.	*Escherichia coli*. a gram-negative, facultative anaerobic, rod-shaped, coliform bacterium commonly found in the lower intestines. When ingested, *E. coli* can cause food poisoning.
EBV.	Epstein-Barr virus is a member of the herpes family known to cause glandular fever as well as various other malignant and non-malignant diseases.

Term	Meaning
embryo.	The early developmental stage within the uterus of the mother—relating to the unborn child until the end of the seventh week following conception; from the eighth week, the unborn child is called a foetus.
EMF.	Electromagnetic frequencies of electromagnetic radiation that propagate energy and travel through space in the form of waves. X-rays and CT-scans but also power lines, mobile phones, microwaves, Wi-Fi routers, computers, and other appliances send out a stream of invisible energy waves. Electric and magnetic fields (EMFs) are produced anywhere electricity is used, including at home and in the workplace. https://lifeenergysolutions.com/street-lamps-with-5g-technology-causing-insomnia-nosebleeds-and-stillbirths/
endocrine glands.	Pineal gland, pituitary gland, pancreas, ovaries, testes, thyroid gland, parathyroid gland, hypothalamus, and adrenal glands. (The pituitary gland and the hypothalamus are neuroendocrine glands.)
epiphyses.	Rounded end of a long bone such as the femur in the leg. Stippled epiphyses is a pattern of focal bone calcification seen in the condition known as chondro-dysplasia punctata. It is caused by use of warfarin, alcohol, and in hypothyroidism.
epithelium.	The "skin" forming the covering of most internal and external surfaces of the human body.
eustachian tube.	Is a hollow tube connecting the middle ear with the nasopharynx, equalising air pressure on both sides of the tympanic membrane (eardrum). It is lined with hair-like projections (cilia) that sweep mucus away from the middle ear towards the nasopharynx.
foetus.	The developing young in the uterus from the end of the eighth week of gestation to the moment of birth.
free radical.	An especially reactive atom or group of atoms that has one or more unpaired electrons. More particularly, a free radical is a reactive atom or group of atoms that is produced in the body by natural biological processes or introduced from an outside source (such as tobacco smoke, toxins, or pollutants) and that can damage cells, proteins, and DNA by altering their chemical structure.

Term	Meaning
gastroschisis.	Internal organs forming outside the body during foetal development.
gene expression.	The process by which the information encoded in a gene is turned into a function. Gene expression can be thought of as an "on/off switch" to control when and where RNA molecules and proteins are made and as a "volume control" to determine how much of those products are made. The process of gene expression is carefully regulated, changing substantially under different conditions and cell types.
GLA.	Gamma linoleic acid, a fatty acid found primarily in seed oils.
glyphosate.	Glyphosate, a broad-spectrum systemic herbicide and crop desiccant. It is an organophosphorus compound.
GMO.	A genetically modified organism. GMOs are organisms (plants, animals, or microorganisms) in which the genetic material (DNA) has been altered in a way that does not occur naturally by mating and/or natural recombination by adding DNA from another species, for example, bacteria.
gonads.	The sex gland, or reproductive gland, is a mixed gland that produces the gametes and sex hormones of an organism. Female reproductive cells are egg cells, and male reproductive cells are sperm. The male gonad, the testicle, produces sperm in the form of spermatozoa. The female gonad, the ovary, produces egg cells.
haematopoiesis.	Formation of red blood cells (in the bone marrow).
HbA1c.	A blood test that shows what your average blood sugar (glucose) level was over the past two to three months.
HHV.	Human herpes virus. HHV includes herpes simplex 1 and 2 and zoster, which causes chicken pox and shingles.
HPV.	Human papilloma virus. HPV belongs to the papilloma virus family.
HTMA.	Hair tissue mineral analysis. Human hair has been accepted as an effective tissue for biological monitoring of toxic heavy metals by the US Environmental Protection Agency and is being used for this purpose throughout the world.

Term	Meaning
hydrocephalus.	A condition in which excess cerebrospinal fluid (CSF) builds up within the fluid-containing cavities or ventricles of the brain. The term "hydrocephalus" is derived from the Greek words "hydro," meaning water, and "cephalus," meaning the head. Although it translates as "water on the brain," the word actually refers to the build-up of cerebrospinal fluid, a clear organic liquid that surrounds the brain and spinal cord.
hydrogenated fats.	Hydrogenation is a process where manufacturers add hydrogen to a liquid fat, such as vegetable oil, to turn it into a solid fat at room temperature. One use of hydrogenated oil is to preserve the shelf life of food. Partially hydrogenated oil contains trans-fat that can raise cholesterol and result in health complications.
hypoxia.	Lack of or insufficient oxygen supply to cells, tissues, or organs.
infertility.	The failure of a couple to conceive a pregnancy after trying to do so for at least one full year. In primary infertility, pregnancy has never occurred. In secondary infertility, one or both members of the couple have previously conceived but are unable to conceive again after a full year of trying.
iridology.	The study of the eye and how the body's physical conditions manifest in the structure of the iris.
MSG.	Monosodium glutamate, a flavour enhancer often added to restaurant foods, canned vegetables, soups, deli meats, and other foods. Glutamate has been linked to neurotoxicity.
myelin.	A lipid (fat)-rich material that surrounds nerve fibres to insulate them and increase the rate of electrical impulses. The myelinated axon can be likened to an electrical wire with insulating material around it. Myelination is the process of creating this insulating fat layer surrounding nerve fibres.
neurilemmal sheath.	Outermost layer of nerve fibres.
neuronal or neurological.	To do with nerves, the central nervous system, and the brain.

Term	Meaning
NPE.	Nonylphenols and nonylphenol ethoxylates—non-ionic surfactants, or detergent-like substances, with uses that lead to widespread release into aquatic environments. They are produced in large volumes and are used for industrial processes and in consumer laundry detergents, personal hygiene, automotive and latex paints, and lawn care products.
NSAIDs.	Non-steroidal anti-inflammatory drugs—members of a therapeutic drug class that reduces pain, decreases inflammation, decreases fever, and prevents blood clots. Side effects depend on the specific drug and its dose and duration of use, but largely include an increased risk of gastrointestinal ulcers and bleeds, heart attack, and kidney disease.
Nutrigenomics.	The science of how nutrition impacts our genome—effectively, how food communicates with your genes.
obesogens.	Foreign chemical compounds hypothesised to disrupt normal development and balance of lipid metabolism, which, in some cases, can lead to obesity.
oocytes.	An immature ovum or female egg cell. An oocyte is produced in a female foetus in the ovary during female gametogenesis.
ovum.	Plural ova—in human physiology, the single cell released from either of the female reproductive organs, the ovaries, which is capable of developing into a new organism when fertilised with a sperm cell.
oxidative damage/ stress.	A consequence of exposure to ionising radiation and a variety of chemical agents and as by-products of normal cellular metabolism. These agents introduce a large number of modifications to DNA.
PAH.	A group of over 100 different chemicals produced during the incomplete burning of fuels, garbage, or other organic substances such as tobacco, plant material, or meats. Studies using pregnant mice fed a specific PAH known as benzo[a]pyrene showed that PAHs may interfere with pregnancy.

Term	Meaning
parenchyma.	The essential or functional elements of an organ, as distinguished from that organ's structure; the specific cells of a gland or organ, contained in and supported by the connective tissue framework.
PBDEs.	Polybrominated diphenyl ethers—a class of organobromine compounds used as flame retardants. The health hazards of these chemicals have attracted increasing scrutiny, and they have been shown to reduce fertility in humans at levels found in households.
PCB.	Polychlorinated biphenyls—any of a class of aromatic organic compounds formed by the chlorination of the hydrocarbon biphenyl. PCBs have many industrial applications but are damaging to the environment. They are highly carcinogenic chemical compounds, formerly used in industrial and consumer products—known carcinogens, classified as persistent organic pollutants (POPs); toxic effects include endocrine disruption and neurotoxicity.
PCOS.	Polycystic ovarian syndrome.
pericardial cavity.	The pericardium—a protective, fluid-filled sac that surrounds the heart and helps it function properly. The pericardium also covers the roots of the major blood vessels as they extend from the heart.
peritoneum.	A continuous membrane that lines the abdominal cavity and covers the abdominal organs (abdominal viscera).
PFCs.	Perfluorinated compounds. PFCs and their derivatives are man-made chemicals that have been used in a wide range of products, including garments and textiles, fabric protection, furniture, and some types of firefighting foam.
PFOA.	Perfluorooctanoic acid. A synthetic, stable perfluorinated carboxylic acid and fluoro surfactant with industrial applications, PFOA is a toxicant and carcinogen in animals, persistent in the environment and associated with infertility.
phthalate.	Any of a group of esters of phthalic acid that are widely used in the manufacture of plastics and as synthetic additives in perfumes and cosmetics. These chemicals have been linked to reproductive and hormonal abnormalities in animals, including humans.

Term	Meaning
plasticity.	A process that involves adaptive structural and functional changes to the brain, nervous tissues, or cells of the body.
pleural cavity.	A fluid-filled space that surrounds the lungs. The pleural cavity is found in the thorax, separating the lungs from its surrounding structures, such as the thoracic cage and intercostal spaces, the mediastinum, and the diaphragm. The pleural cavity is bounded by a double-layered serous membrane called pleura.
POPs.	Persistent organic pollutants—toxic chemicals that adversely affect human health and the environment around the world. Because they can be transported by wind and water, most POPs generated in one country can and do affect people and wildlife far from where they are used and released. They persist for long periods of time in the environment and can accumulate and pass from one species to the next through the food chain.
prostaglandins.	Potent hormone-like substances produced in various mammalian tissues. Derived from arachidonic acid, prostaglandins mediate a wide range of physiological functions, such as control of blood pressure, contraction of smooth muscle, and modulation of inflammation.
Pulmonary hypertension.	Increased blood pressure in the arteries of the lungs.
seminal fluid.	Another term for semen. Seminal fluid is emitted from the male reproductive tract and contains sperm cells, which are capable of fertilising the female's eggs. Semen also contains liquids that combine to form seminal plasma, which helps keep the sperm cells viable.
SOD.	Superoxide dismutase is an enzyme that breaks down the superoxide radical into ordinary molecular oxygen and hydrogen peroxide. Superoxide is produced as a by-product of oxygen metabolism and, if not regulated, causes many types of cell damage.
teratogen.	Any agent or substance that can cause malformation of an embryo or birth defects or that interferes with normal embryonic development—alcohol or thalidomide or X-rays or rubella are examples.

Term	Meaning
trans-fats/trans-fatty acids/TFAs.	Manufactured TFAs (also known as artificial TFAs) are formed when liquid vegetable oils are partially hydrogenated or "hardened" during processing to create spreads such as margarine, cooking fats for deep-frying, and shortening for baking. Some TFAs are also formed during high-temperature cooking. There is strong evidence that TFAs increase the amount of "bad" low-density lipoprotein (LDL) cholesterol in our blood, a major risk factor for coronary heart disease.
transglutaminase.	Any of a family of enzymes that catalyse the reaction of lysine and glutamine groups in proteins and have a function in blood coagulation. Transglutaminas are used in meat, fish, dairy, and bakery products.
tympanic membrane.	Eardrum.
utero.	Uterus, womb.
ventricular septal defect.	A hole in the heart. A VSD is a common heart problem present at birth (congenital heart defect). The hole occurs in the wall that separates the heart's lower chambers (ventricles).
viscera.	The soft internal organs of the body, especially those contained within the abdominal and thoracic cavities—specifically those within the chest (as the heart or lungs) or abdomen (as the liver, pancreas, or intestines).

ACKNOWLEDGEMENTS

This book could not have happened without the inspiration from my daughter, as well as the unwavering support and patience of my wonderful husband.

I'd like to thank all my patients who have come to see me since I opened my first clinic in 2000 and for allowing me to be a part of your healing journeys. I've learned so much from you all.

Thank you to Bianka and Erin for taking the time to read my draft manuscript, providing valuable feedback and suggestions, and allowing me to share their personal experiences of motherhood. Thanks also to Natalie for permitting me to share her story.

To all the lecturers at the colleges and university I studied at who encouraged and supported my passion for natural medicine, thank you for nurturing my need to find answers. In particular, thank you to Mark A. Nicholson, ASO, for challenging us to always look beyond the obvious.

To the scholars and educators both here in Australia and overseas for their ongoing research and sharing of knowledge, as well as unwavering dedication to natural, integrative, and functional medicine.

PERMISSIONS

Table 1. Embryonic timeline
https://embryology.med.unsw.edu.au/embryology/index.php/Timeline_-_human development
Cite this page: Hill, M.A. (2023, February 8) Embryology, Abnormal Development—Teratogens. Retrieved from https://embryology.med.unsw.edu.au/embryology/index.php/Abnormal Development - Teratogens
Dr Mark Hill 2023, UNSW Embryology ISBN: 978 0 7334 2609 4—UNSW CRICOS Provider Code No. 00098G

Table 2. Diagram of gut health—G.E.M.M. Dr Christine Houghton. Image credit: Gut-Immune Response; Dr Christine Houghton, Nutrigenomic Medicine, https://nutrigenomicmedicine.com/.

Food pyramids. No modifications were made to the image, and the original credit/copyright notice line was included.

The poem "**Desiderata.**" In 1975, the court ruled and subsequently the Seventh Circuit Court of Appeals upheld) that copyright had been abandoned and forfeited because the poem had been authorised for publication without a copyright notice in 1933 and 1942—and that the poem was therefore in the public domain.

The quote used as the chapter 16 epigraph, "Investing in early childhood nutrition is a surefire strategy. The re turns are in credibly high." (Anne M. Mulcahy) was sourced from https://stresslessbehealthy.com/healthy-eating-quotes/.

SOURCES AND REFERENCES

All links were active during the time of writing this book.
However, ongoing access cannot be guaranteed.

1. "The Top Three Reasons Infertility Is on the Rise," Genea Fertility, SA, January 11, 2018, https://fertilitysa.com.au/2018/01/11/the-top-3-reasons-fertility-is-on-the-rise.
2. AIHW, "Poor Diet," Australian Institute of Health and Welfare website, July 18, 2019, https://www.aihw.gov.au/reports/food-nutrition/poor-diet/contents/poor-diet-in-adults.
3. https://www.sciencedirect.com/topics/materials-science/oxidative-damage
4. A. Agarwal, S. Roychoudhury, R. Sharma, S. Gupta, A. Majzoub, and E. Sabanegh, "Diagnostic Application of Oxidation-Reduction Potential Assay for Measurement of Oxidative Stress: Clinical Utility in Male Factor Infertility, *Reprod Biomed Online* 34, no. 1, (January 2017): 48–57, doi: 10.1016/j.rbmo.2016.10.008, epub October 20, 2016, PMID: 27839743.
5. https://www.fertility.com.au/.
6. https://www.abc.net.au/health/library/stories/2007/05/30/1919840.htm.
7. M. B.Sørensen, I .A. Bergdahl, N. H. Hjøllund, J. P. Bonde, M. Stoltenberg, and E Ernst, "Zinc, Magnesium and Calcium in Human Seminal Fluid: Relations to Other Semen Parameters and Fertility," *Molecular Human Reproduction* 5, no. 4 (April 1999): 331–37, https://doi.org/10.1093/molehr/5.4.331. M. Tikkiwal et al, "Effect of Zinc Administration on Seminal Zinc and Fertility of Oligospermic Males," *Ind J Phys Pharm* 31 (1987):30–34, https://ijpp.com/IJPP%20archives/1987_31_1/30-34.pdf
8. G. Danscher et al., "Zinc Content of Human Ejaculate and the Motility of Sperm Cells," *Int J Androl* 1 (1978): 576–81, https://onlinelibrary.wiley.com/doi/pdf/10.1111/j.1365-2605.1978.tb00628.x.
9. O. Akinloye et al, "Selenium Status of Idiopathic Infertile Nigerian Males," *Biological Trace Element Research* 104 (2005): 9–18.
10. H. J. Chi, J. H. Kim, C. S. Ryu, J. Y. Lee, J. S. Park, D.Y. Chung, S. Y. Choi, M. H. Kim, E. K. Chun, and S. I. Roh, "Protective Effect of Antioxidant Supplementation in Sperm-Preparation Medium against Oxidative Stress in Human Spermatozoa," *Hum Reprod* 23, no. 5 (May 2008): 1023–8, doi: 10.1093/humrep/den060, epub March 5, 2008, PMID: 18325884.
11. R. Scott, A. MacPherson, R. W. Yates, B. Hussain, and J Dixon, "The Effect of oral Selenium Supplementation on Human Sperm Motility," *Br J Urol* 82, no. 1 (July 1998): 76–80, doi: 10.1046/j.1464-410x.1998.00683.x. PMID: 9698665.

12 A. T. Alahmar, A. E. Calogero, R. Singh, R. Cannarella, P. Sengupta, and S. Dutta, "Coenzyme Q10, Oxidative Stress, and Male Infertility: A review," *Clinical and Experimental Reproductive Medicine* 48 no. 2 (2021): 97–104, https://doi.org/10.5653/cerm.2020.04175.
13 https://imb.uq.edu.au/article/2004/05/scientists-tackle-decline-male-fertility.
14 H. Levine, N. Jørgensen, A. Martino-Andrade, J. Mendiola, D. Weksler-Derri, I. Mindlis, R. Pinotti, and S. H. Swan, "Temporal Trends in Sperm Count: A Systematic Review and Meta-Regression Analysis," *Hum Reprod Update* 23, no. 6 (November 1, 2017): 646–59, doi: 10.1093/humupd/dmx022, PMID: 28981654, PMCID: PMC6455044.
15 M. N. Mead, "Nutrigenomics: The Genome—Food Interface," *Environ Health Perspect* 115, no. 12 (December 2007): A582–9, doi: 10.1289/ehp.115-a582, PMID: 18087577, PMCID: PMC2137135.
16 F. Sciarra, E. Franceschini, F. Campolo, D. Gianfrilli, F. Pallotti, D. Paoli, A.M. Isidori and M. A. Venneri, "Disruption of Circadian Rhythms: A Crucial Factor in the Etiology of Infertility," *International Journal of Molecular Sciences*, 21, no. 11 (2020), https://doi.org/10.3390/ijms21113943.
17 https://techwellness.com/blogs/expertise/laptop-rf-radiation-danger-protection-from-emf.
18 A. Agarwal, S. Roychoudhury, R. Sharma, S. Gupta, A. Majzoub, and E. Sabanegh, "Diagnostic Application of Oxidation-Reduction Potential Assay for Measurement of Oxidative Stress: Clinical Utility in Male Factor Infertility," *Reprod Biomed Online* 34, no. 1 (January 2017): 48–57, doi: 10.1016/j.rbmo.2016.10.008, epub October 20, 2016, PMID: 27839743.
19 Agarwal et al., "Diagnostic Application of Oxidation-Reduction."
20 Dr Stephanie Seneff, PhD, *Toxic Legacy: How the Weedkiller Glyphosate Is Destroying Our Health and the Environment*, (Vermont: Chelsea Green).
21 Seneff, *Toxic Legacy*.
22 A. Cherskov, A. Pohl, C. Allison, H. Zhang, R. A. Payne, and S. Baron-Cohen, "Polycystic Ovary Syndrome and Autism: A Test of the Prenatal Sex Steroid Theory, *Transl Psychiatry* 8, no. 1 (August 1, 2018): 136, doi: 10.1038/s41398-018-0186-7, PMID: 30065244, PMCID: PMC6068102.
23 R. Koedooder, M. Singer, S. Schoenmakers, P. H. M. Savelkoul, S. A. Morré, J. D. de Jonge, L. Poort, W. J. S. S. Cuypers, N. G. M. Beckers, F. J. M. Broekmans, B. J. Cohlen, J. E. den Hartog, K. Fleischer, C. B. Lambalk, J. M. J. S. Smeenk, A. E. Budding, and J. S. E. Laven, "The Vaginal Microbiome as a Predictor for Outcome of In Vitro Fertilization with or without Intracytoplasmic Sperm Injection: A Prospective Study," *Hum Reprod* 34, no. 6 (June 2019): 1,042–54, doi: 10.1093/humrep/dez065. Erratum in *Hum Reprod* 34, no. 10 (October 2, 2019): 2,091–92, PMID: 31119299.

24　J. D. Kloss, M. L. Perlis, J. A. Zamzow, E. J. Culnan, and C. R. Gracia, "Sleep, Sleep Disturbance, and Fertility in Women," *Sleep Medicine Reviews* 22 (2015): 78–87, https://doi.org/10.1016/j.smrv.2014.10.005.

25　K. Van Heertum and B. Rossi, "Alcohol and Fertility: How Much Is Too Much?" *Fertility Research and Practice* 3 (2017): 10, https://doi.org/10.1186/s40738-017-0037-x.

26　https://childrenshealthdefense.org/news/infant-and-child-mortality-in-the-u-s-nothing-to-brag-about/.

27　Dr Mark Donohoe, "Link between Parents Toxicity and Children's Behavioural Disorders," https://www.youtube.com/watch?v=cm08EZH02Zw -.

28　https://truemedicine.com.au/tips/good-health-starts-in-the-mouth/.

29　M. A. Hill, M.A. "Embryology Human-Critical Periods of Development," March 20, 2023, retrieved from https://embryology.med.unsw.edu.au/embryology/index.php/File:Human-critical_periods_of_development.jpg.

30　M. A. Hill, "Embryology Abnormal Development—Teratogens," February 8, 2023, retrieved from https://embryology.med.unsw.edu.au/embryology/index.php/Abnormal_Development_-_Teratogens.

31　American Chemical Society National Historic Chemical Landmarks, Chemical Abstracts Service (CAS), accessed January 2023, http://www.acs.org/content/acs/en/education/whatischemistry/landmarks/cas.html.

32　Department of Agriculture, "Water and the Environment. Chemicals of Concern in Plastics," accessed February 10, 2023, https://www.awe.gov.au/environment/protection/chemicals-management/chemicals-of-concern-plastics.

33　I. Dubey, S. Khan, and S. Kushwaha, "Developmental and Reproductive Toxic Effects of Exposure to Microplastics: A Review of Associated Signalling Pathways," *Frontiers in Toxicology* 4 (2022), 901798, https://doi.org/10.3389/ftox.2022.901798.

34　W. J. Crinnion, "Toxic Effects of the Easily Avoidable Phthalates and Parabens," *Altern Med Rev* 15, no. 3 (September 2010): 190–6, PMID: 21155623.

35　H. Hlisníková, I. Petrovičová, B. Kolena, M. Šidlovská, and A. Sirotkin, "Effects and Mechanisms of Phthalates Action on Reproductive Processes and Reproductive Health: A Literature Review," *International Journal of Environmental Research and Public Health* 17, no. 18 (2020), https://doi.org/10.3390/ijerph17186811.

36　A. Konieczna, A. Rutkowska, and D. Rachoń, "Health Risk of Exposure to Bisphenol A (BPA)," *Rocz Panstw Zakl Hig* 66, no. 1 (2015) :5–11, PMID: 25813067.

37　A. Ragusa, A. Svelato, C. Santacroce et al., "Plasticenta: First Evidence of Microplastics in Human Placenta," *Environ Int* 146 (2021): 106,274, doi:10.1016/j.envint.2020.106274.

38 C. Campanale, C. Massarelli, I. Savino, V. Locaputo, and V. F. Uricchio, "A Detailed Review Study on Potential Effects of Microplastics and Additives of Concern on Human Health," Int J Environ Res Public Health 17, no. 4 (2020), doi:10.3390/ijerph17041212.

39 https://truemedicine.com.au/treatments/childrens-health/autism-spectrum-disorders/brain-inflammation/.

40 G. B. Post, P. D. Cohn, and K. R. Cooper, "Perfluorooctanoic Acid (PFOA), an Emerging Drinking Water Contaminant: A Critical Review of recent Literature," Environ Res 116 (July 2012): 93–117, doi: 10.1016/j.envres.2012.03.007, epub May 4, 2012, PMID: 22560884.

41 S. Rajender, K. Avery, and A. Agarwal, "Epigenetics, Spermatogenesis and Male Infertility," Mutat Res 727, no. 3 (May–June 2011): 62–71, doi: 10.1016/j.mrrev.2011.04.002, epub April 16, 2011, PMID: 21540125.

42 A. Soares, B. Guieysse, B. Jefferson, E. Cartmell, and J. N. Lester, "Nonylphenol in the Environment: A Critical Review on Occurrence, Fate, Toxicity and Treatment in Wastewaters," Environ Int 34, no. 7 (October 2008): 1,033–49, doi: 10.1016/j.envint.2008.01.004, epub February 20, 2008, PMID: 18282600.

43 W. J. Pizzi, J. E. Barnhart, and D.J. Fanslow, "Monosodium Glutamate Administration to the Newborn Reduces Reproductive Ability in Female and Male Mice," Science 196, no. 4288 (April 22, 1977): 452–4, doi: 10.1126/science.557837, PMID: 557837 (fertility); R. P. Biney, F. T. Djankpa, S. A. Osei, D. L. Egbenya, B. Aboagye, A. A. Karikari, A. Ussif, G. A. Wiafe, and D. Nuertey, "Effects of In Utero Exposure to Monosodium Glutamate on locomotion, Anxiety, Depression, Memory and KCC2 Expression in Offspring, Int J Dev Neurosci 82, no. 1 (February 2022): 50–62, doi: 10.1002/jdn.10158, epub December 1, 2021, PMID: 34755371 (neurological disorders).

44 https://www.hsph.harvard.edu/magazine/magazine article/fluoridated-drinking-water/.

45 https://takecontrol.substack.com/p/biomilq-fake-milk.

46 H. Levine, N. Jørgensen, A. Martino-Andrade, J. Mendiola, D. Weksler-Derri, I. Mindlis, R. Pinotti, and S. H. Swan, "Temporal Trends in Sperm Count: A Systematic Review and Meta-Regression Analysis," Hum Reprod Update 23, no. 6 (November 1, 2017): 646–59, doi: 10.1093/humupd/dmx022, PMID: 28981654, PMCID: PMC6455044.

47 G. Arya, S. Tadayon, J. Sadighian, J. Jones, K. de Mutsert, T. B. Huff, and G. D. Foster, "Pharmaceutical Chemicals, Steroids and Xenoestrogens in Water, Sediments and Fish from the Tidal Freshwater Potomac River (Virginia, USA)," J Environ Sci Health A Tox Hazard Subst Environ Eng 52, no. 7 (June 7, 2017): 686–96, doi: 10.1080/10934529.2017.1312975, epub April 27, 2017, PMID: 28448746.

48 Australian Bureau of Statistics (ABS), "National Health Survey: Summary of Results 2004–2005," 2006, accessed September 30, 2007, from http://www.abs.gov.au.
49 K. L. Moore and T.V.N. Persaud, *The Developing Human: Clinically Oriented Embryology* (Philadelphia: Saunders, 2003).
50 F. Burdan and A. Bełzek, "Współczesne poglady na embriotoksyczne i teratogenne działanie ibuprofenu" ("Current Opinions on Embryotoxic and Teratogenic Effects of Ibuprofen"), *Pol Merkur Lekarski* 11, no. 63 (September 2001): 266–70, Polish, PMID: 11761827.
51 C. P. Torfs, E. A. Katz, T. F. Bateson, P. K. Lam, and C. J. Curry. "Maternal Medications and Environmental Exposures as Risk Factors for Gastroschisis, *Teratology* 54, no. 2 (August 1996): 84–92, doi: 10.1002/(SICI)1096-9926(199606)54:2<84::AID-TERA4>3.0.CO;2-4. PMID: 8948544.
52 F. Burdan, "Ocena bezpieczeństwa stosowania kwasu acetylosalicylowego w okresie prenatalnym" ("Prenatal Effects of Acetylsalicylic Acid"), *Pol Merkur Lekarski* 11, no. 62 (August 2001): 182–6, Polish, PMID: 11757226.
53 B. Ofori, D. Oraichi, L. Blais, E. Rey, and A. Bérard, "Risk of Congenital Anomalies in Pregnant Users of Non-Steroidal Anti-Inflammatory Drugs: A Nested Case-Control Study," *Birth Defects Res B Dev Reprod Toxicol* 77, no. 4 (August 2006): 268–79, doi: 10.1002/bdrb.20085, PMID: 16929547.
54 R. Stahlmann, and S. Klug, eds., *Antiviral Agents. Drug Toxicity in Embryonic Development ll—Advances in Understanding Mechanisms of Birth Defects: Mechanistics Understanding of Human Development Toxicants* (Berlin: Springer, 1997).
55 https://childrenshealthdefense.org/news/infant-and-child-mortality-in-the-u-s-nothing-to-brag-about/.
56 https://www.tga.gov.au/products/medicines/find-information-about-medicine/prescribing-medicines-pregnancy-database.
57 M. M. Iqbal, T. Sobhan, and T. Ryals, "Effects of Commonly Used Benzodiazepines on the Fetus, the Neonate, and the Nursing Infant," *Psychiatr Serv* 53, no. 1 (January 2002): 39–49, doi: 10.1176/appi.ps.53.1.39. PMID: 11773648.
58 E. Jauniaux, D. Jurkovic, C. Lees, S. Campbell, and B Gulbis, "In-Vivo Study of Diazepam Transfer across the First Trimester Human Placenta," *Hum Reprod* 11, no. 4 (April 1996): 889–92, doi: 10.1093/oxfordjournals.humrep.a019272, PMID: 8671346.
59 A. Bérard, E. Ramos, E. Rey, L. Blais, M. St-André, and D. Oraichi, "First Trimester Exposure to Paroxetine and Risk of Cardiac Malformations in Infants: The Importance of Dosage," B*irth Defects Res B Dev Reprod Toxicol* 80, no. 1 (February 2007): 18–27, doi: 10.1002/bdrb.20099, PMID: 17187388.

60 M. M. Iqbal, S. P. Gundlapalli, W. G. Ryan, T. Ryals, and T. E. Passman, "Effects of Antimanic Mood-Stabilizing Drugs on Fetuses, Neonates, and Nursing Infants," *South Med J.* 94, no. 3 (March 2001): 304–22, PMID: 11284518.

61 M. Narang, D. Shah, and G. Natasha, "Intracranial Arteriovenous Malformation with Maternal Carbamazepine Use," *Indian J Pediatr* 74, no. 1 (January 2007): 85–6, doi: 10.1007/s12098-007-0035-9, PMID: 17264463.

62 https://truemedicine.com.au/health-tips/nutrition-digestion-health/gord-gastro-oesophageal-reflux-disease/.

63 J. M. Rogers and G. P. Daston, eds., *Alcohols: Ethanol and Methanol. Drug Toxicity in Embryonic Development ll* (Berlin: Springer, 1997).

64 J. P. Newnham, T. J. Moss, I. Nitsos, D. M. Sloboda, and J. R. Challis, "Nutrition and the Early Origins of Adult Disease," *Asia Pac J Clin Nutr* 11, suppl. 3 (2002): S537–42, doi: 10.1046/j.1440-6047.11.supp3.11.x, PMID: 12492645.

65 E. Villamor and W. W. Fawzi, "Effects of Vitamin a Supplementation on Immune Responses and Correlation with Clinical Outcomes," *Clin Microbiol Rev* 18, no. 3 (July 2005): 446–64, doi: 10.1128/CMR.18.3.446-464.2005, PMID: 16020684, PMCID: PMC1195969.

66 R.J. Kavlock and G. P. Daston, eds., *Drug Toxicity in Embryonic Development ll* (Berlin: Springer-Verlag, 1997).

67 U. Kapil, "Impact of Single /Multiple Micronutrient Supplementation on Child Health," *Indian J Pediatr* 71, no. 11 (November 2004): 983–4, doi: 10.1007/BF02828112, PMID: 15572817.

68 V. Azaïs-Braesco and G. Pascal, "Vitamin A in Pregnancy: Requirements and Safety Limits," *Am J Clin Nutr* 71, suppl. 5 (May 2000): 1,325S–33S, doi: 10.1093/ajcn/71.5.1325s, PMID: 10799410.

69 https://www.boisestate.edu/undergraduate-research/2020/04/22/186-methodology-to-assess-effects-environmental-toxins-on-reproductive-health/.

70 D. Raubenheimer and S. J. Simpson, *Eat Like the Animals: What Nature Teaches Us about the Science of Healthy Eating* (New York: Harper Collins, 2020).

71 https://www.livestrong.com/article/272066-why-is-hydrogenated-oil-bad-for-you/.

72 https://lpi.oregonstate.edu/mic/other-nutrients/essential-fatty-acids#pregnancy-early-childhood-developmental-outcomes.

73 S. E. Carlson, J. Colombo, B. J. Gajewski, K. M. Gustafson, D. Mundy, J. Yeast, M. K. Georgieff, L. A. Markley, E. H. Kerling, and D. J. Shaddy, "DHA Supplementation and Pregnancy Outcomes," *Am J Clin Nutr* 97, no. 4 (April 2013): 808–15, doi: 10.3945/ajcn.112.050021, epub February 20, 2013, PMID: 23426033, PMCID: PMC3607655.

74 R. K. McNamara, J. Able, R. Jandacek, T. Rider, P. Tso, J. C. Eliassen, D. Alfieri, W. Weber, K. Jarvis, M. P. DelBello, S. M. Strakowski, and C. M. Adler, "Docosahexaenoic Acid Supplementation Increases Prefrontal Cortex Activation

during Sustained Attention in Healthy Boys: A Placebo-Controlled, Dose-Ranging, Functional Magnetic Resonance Imaging Study," *Am J Clin Nutr* 91, no. 4 (April 2010): 1,060–7, doi: 10.3945/ajcn.2009.28549, epub February 3, 2010, PMID: 20130094, PMCID: PMC2844685.

75 C. Y. Chang, D. S. Ke, and J. Y. Chen, "Essential Fatty Acids and Human Brain," *Acta Neurol Taiwan* 18, no. 4 (December 2009): 231–41, PMID: 20329590.

76 S. H. Zeisel, "Choline: Critical Role during Fetal Development and Dietary Requirements in Adults," *Annu Rev Nutr* 26 (2006): 229–50, doi: 10.1146/annurev.nutr.26.061505.111156, PMID: 16848706, PMCID: PMC2441939.

77 A. M. Mahmoud and M. M. Ali, "Methyl Donor Micronutrients that Modify DNA Methylation and Cancer Outcome," *Nutrients* 11, no. 3 (March 2019): 608, doi: 10.3390/nu11030608, PMID: 30871166, PMCID: PMC6471069.

78 M. D. Niculescu and S. H. Zeisel, "Diet, Methyl Donors and DNA Methylation: Interactions between Dietary Folate, Methionine and Choline," *J Nutr* 132, suppl. 8 (August 2002): 2,333S–35S), doi: 10.1093/jn/132.8.2333S, PMID: 12163687.

79 N. S. Wadhwani, V. V. Patil, S. S. Mehendale, G. N. Wagh, S. A. Gupte, and S. R. Joshi, "Increased Homocysteine Levels Exist in Women with Preeclampsia from Early Pregnancy," *J Matern Fetal Neonatal Med* 29, no. 16 (2016): 2,719–25, doi: 10.3109/14767058.2015.1102880, epub November 9, 2015, PMID: 26552939 (preeclampsia); W. L. Nelen, H. J. Blom, E. A. Steegers, M. den Heijer, and T. K. Eskes, "Hyperhomocysteinemia and Recurrent Early Pregnancy Loss: A Meta-Analysis," *Fertil Steril* 74, no. 6 (December 2000): 1,196–9, doi: 10.1016/s0015-0282(00)01595-8, PMID: 11119750 (miscarriage).

80 https://www.bluezones.com/2020/07/blue-zones-diet-food-secrets-of-the-worlds-longest-lived-people/.

81 A. Crimarco, M. J. Landry, M. M. Carter, and C. D. Gardner, "Assessing the Effects of Alternative Plant-Based Meats v. Animal Meats on Biomarkers of Inflammation: A Secondary Analysis of the SWAP-MEAT Randomized Crossover Trial, *J Nutr Sci* 11 (September 23, 2022): e82, doi: 10.1017/jns.2022.84, PMID: 36304815, PMCID: PMC9554424.

82 https://truemedicine.com.au/tips/want-to-adopt-a-vegan-diet/.

83 https://chemicalmaze.com/.

84 https://truemedicine.com.au/wp-content/uploads/meal_planning.PDF.

85 H. H. Hermsdorff, M. A. Zulet, B. Puchau, and J. A. Martínez, "Fruit and Vegetable Consumption and Proinflammatory Gene Expression from Peripheral Blood Mononuclear Cells in Young Adults: A Translational Study," *Nutr Metab (Lond)* 7 (May 13, 2010): 42, doi: 10.1186/1743-7075-7-42, PMID: 20465828, PMCID: PMC2882916.

86 A. Lerner and T. Matthias, "Changes in Intestinal Tight Junction Permeability Associated with Industrial Food Additives Explain the Rising Incidence of

Autoimmune Disease," Elsevier 2015, https://www.sciencedirect.com/science/article/pii/S1568997215000245 https://doi.org/10.1016/j.autrev.2015.01.009.

87 Russell L. Blaylock, *Excitotoxins: The Taste that Kills* (Santa Fe: Health Press).

88 Dr Christine Houghton, *Switched On: Harnessing the Power of Nutrigenomics to Optimise Your Health* (Brisbane: Integra Publishing), https://nutrigenomicmedicine.com/.

89 S. Wang, K. Zhang, Y. Yao, J. Li, and S. Deng, "Bacterial Infections Affect Male Fertility: A Focus on the Oxidative Stress-Autophagy Axis," *Front Cell Dev Biol* 9 (October 21, 2021): 727,812, doi: 10.3389/fcell.2021.727812, PMID: 34746124, PMCID: PMC8566953.

90 A. Lerner and T. Matthias, "Changes in Intestinal Tight Junction Permeability Associated with Industrial Food Additives Explain the Rising Incidence of Autoimmune Disease," *Autoimmun Rev* 14, no. 6 (June 2015): 479–89, doi: 10.1016/j.autrev.2015.01.009, epub February 9, 2015, PMID: 25676324.

91 https://www.totalhealth.co.uk/blog/alcohol-converts-acetaldehyde-and-can-cause-cancer.

92 C. H. Ramlau-Hansen, G. Toft, M. S. Jensen, K. Strandberg-Larsen, M. L. Hansen, and J. Olsen, "Maternal Alcohol Consumption during Pregnancy and Semen Quality in the Male Offspring: Two Decades of Follow-Up," *Hum Reprod* 25, no. 9 (September 2010): 2,340–5, doi: 10.1093/humrep/deq140, epub June 29, 2010, PMID: 20587536.

93 Dr F. Batmanghelidj, http://www.watercure.com/.

94 E. van den Boogaard, R. Vissenberg, J. A. Land, M. van Wely, J. A. van der Post, M. Goddijn, P. H. Bisschop, "Significance of (Sub)Clinical Thyroid Dysfunction and Thyroid Autoimmunity before Conception and in Early Pregnancy: A Systematic Review," *Hum Reprod Update* 17, no. 5 (September–October 2011): 605–19, doi: 10.1093/humupd/dmr024, epub May 28, 2011, erratum in *Hum Reprod Update* 22, no. 4 (June 2016): 532–3, PMID: 21622978.

95 K. M. Gustafson, S. E. Carlson, J. Colombo, H. W. Yeh, D. J. Shaddy, S. Li, and E. H. Kerling, "Effects of Docosahexaenoic Acid Supplementation during Pregnancy on Fetal Heart Rate and Variability: A Randomized Clinical Trial," *Prostaglandins Leukot Essent Fatty Acids* 88, no. 5 (May 2013): 331–8, doi: 10.1016/j.plefa.2013.01.009, epub February 20, 2013, PMID: 23433688, PMCID: PMC3734850.

96 T. Moore, Arefadib, Alana Deery, and Sue West, *The First Thousand Days: An Evidence Paper*, https://www.researchgate.net/publication/320057527 The _ First_Thousand_Days_An Evidence Paper.

97 N. M. Nnam, "Improving Maternal Nutrition for Better Pregnancy Outcomes," *Proc Nutr Soc* 74, no. 4 (November 2015): 454–9, doi: 10.1017/S0029665115002396, epub August 12, 2015, PMID: 26264457.

98 A. J. Whitehouse, B. J. Holt, M. Serralha, P. G. Holt, M. M. Kusel, and P. H. Hart, "Maternal Serum Vitamin D Levels during Pregnancy and Offspring Neurocognitive Development," *Pediatrics* 129, no. 3 (March 2012): 4,854–93, doi: 10.1542/peds.2011-2644, epub February 13, 2012, PMID: 22331333.

99 S. N. Karras, H. Fakhoury, G. Muscogiuri, W. B. Grant, J. M. van den Ouweland, A. M. Colao, and K. Kotsa, "Maternal Vitamin D Levels during Pregnancy and Neonatal Health: Evidence to Date and Clinical Implications, *Ther Adv Musculoskelet Dis* 8, no. 4 (August): 1,244–35, doi: 10.1177/1759720X16656810, epub July 13, 2016, PMID: 27493691, PMCID: PMC4959630.

100 S. Akbari and A. A. Rasouli-Ghahroudi, "Vitamin K and Bone Metabolism: A Review of the Latest Evidence in Preclinical Studies," *Biomed Res Int* (June 27, 2018): 4,629,383, doi: 10.1155/2018/4629383, PMID: 30050932, PMCID: PMC6040265.

101 National Health and Medical Research Council, Manganese [Internet], Canberra (ACT): Australian Government, https://www.nrv.gov.au/nutrients/manganese.

102 L. Braun and M. Cohen, *Herbs and Natural Supplements: An Evidence-Based Guide*, vol. 2, 4th ed. (Sydney: Elsevier/Churchill Livingstone, 2015), 575–83; Health and Medical Research Council, Nutrient Reference Values for Australia and New Zealand, "Iodine" eatforhealth.gov.au website, Canberra (ACT): Australian Government, https://www.eatforhealth.gov.au/nutrient-reference-values/nutrients/iodine.

103 S. A. Skeaff, "Iodine Deficiency in Pregnancy: The Effect on Neurodevelopment in the Child," *Nutrients* 3, no. 2 (February 2011): 265–73, doi: 10.3390/nu3020265, epub February 18, 2011, PMID: 22254096, PMCID: PMC3257674.

104 https://www.fxmedicine.com.au/podcast/intricacies-iodine-rachel-arthur.

105 L. Iglesias, J. Canals, and V. Arija, "Effects of Prenatal Iron Status on Child Neurodevelopment and Behavior: A Systematic Review," *Crit Rev Food Sci Nutr* 58, no. 10 (July 3, 2018): 1,604–14, doi: 10.1080/10408398.2016.1274285, epub June 12, 2017, PMID: 28084782.

106 Henry Osiecki, *The Nutrient Bible*, 7th ed. (Eagle Farm: AG Publishing).

107 N. Melamed, A. Ben-Haroush, B. Kaplan, and Y. Yogev, "Iron Supplementation in Pregnancy: Does the Preparation Matter?" *Arch Gynecol Obstet* 276, no. 6 (December 2007): 601–4, doi: 10.1007/s00404-007-0388-3, epub May 31, 2007, PMID: 17541618.

108 https://truemedicine.com.au/tips/low-iron/.

109 H. M. Baker and E. N. Baker, "Lactoferrin and Iron: Structural and Dynamic Aspects of Binding and Release," *Biometals* 17, no. 3 (June 2004): 209–16, doi: 10.1023/b:biom.0000027694.40260.70, PMID: 15222467.

110 https://www.health.harvard.edu/blog/how-safe-is-exercise-during-pregnancy-2020012818760.

111 S. L. Carmichael, W. Yang, and G. M. Shaw, "Periconceptional Nutrient Intakes and Risks of Neural Tube Defects in California," *Birth Defects Res A Clin Mol Teratol* 88, no. 8 (August 2010): 670–8, doi: 10.1002/bdra.20675, PMID: 20740594, PMCID: PMC2929981.

112 J. M. Petersen, S. E. Parker, K. S. Crider, S. C. Tinker, A. A. Mitchell, and M. M. Werler, "One-Carbon Cofactor Intake and Risk of Neural Tube Defects among Women Who Meet Folic Acid Recommendations: A Multicenter Case-Control Study," *Am J Epidemiol* 188, no. 6 (June 1, 2019): 1,136–43, doi: 10.1093/aje/kwz040, PMID: 30976786, PMCID: PMC6545279.

113 H. J. Blom, G. M. Shaw, M. den Heijer, and R. H. Finnell, "Neural Tube Defects and folate: case far from Closed," *Nat Rev Neurosci* 7, no. 9 (September 2006): 724–31, doi: 10.1038/nrn1986, PMID: 16924261, PMCID: PMC2970514.

114 K. Pietrzik, L. Bailey, and B. Shane, "Folic Acid and L-5-Methyltetrahydrofolate: Comparison of Clinical Pharmacokinetics and Pharmacodynamics," *Clin Pharmacokinet* 49, no. 8 (August 2010): 535–48, doi: 10.2165/11532990-000000000-00000, PMID: 20608755; E. J. Servy, L. Jacquesson-Fournols, M. Cohen, and Y. J. R Menezo, "MTHFR Isoform Carriers. 5-MTHF (5-Methyl Tetrahydrofolate) vs Folic Acid: A Key to Pregnancy Outcome—a Case Series," *J Assist Reprod Genet* 35, no. 8 (August 2018): 1,431–35, doi: 10.1007/s10815-018-1225-2, epub June 7, 2018, PMID: 29882091, PMCID: PMC6086798.

115 S. H. Zeisel, "Nutrition in Pregnancy: The Argument for Including a Source of Choline," *Int J Womens Health* 5 (April 22, 2013): 193–9, doi: 10.2147/IJWH.S36610, PMID: 23637565, PMCID: PMC3639110.

116 M. A. Caudill, B. J. Strupp, L. Muscalu, J. E. H. Nevins, and R. L. Canfield, "Maternal Choline Supplementation during the third Trimester of Pregnancy Improves Infant Information Processing Speed: A Randomized, Double-Blind, Controlled Feeding Study," *FASEB J* 32, no. 4 (April 2018): 2,172–80, doi: 10.1096/fj.201700692RR, epub January 5, 2018, PMID: 29217669, PMCID: PMC6988845.

117 R. Vishwanathan, M. J. Kuchan, S. Sen, and E. J. Johnson, "Lutein and Preterm Infants with Decreased Concentrations of brain Carotenoids," *J Pediatr Gastroenterol Nutr* 59, no. 5 (November 2014): 659–65, doi: 10.1097/MPG.0000000000000389, PMID: 24691400.

118 D. B. Nelson, S. Bellamy, I. Nachamkin, R. B. Ness, G. A. Macones, and L. Allen-Taylor, "First Trimester Bacterial Vaginosis, Individual Microorganism Levels, and Risk of Second Trimester Pregnancy Loss among Urban Women," *Fertil Steril* 88, no. 5 (November 2007): 1,396–403, doi: 10.1016/j.fertnstert.2007.01.035, epub April 16, 2007, PMID: 17434499, PMCID: PMC2094106.

119 M. W. Jones, C. B. Weir, and S. Ghassemzadeh, "Gallstones (Cholelithiasis)," updated October 24, 2022, in StatPearls (internet) (Treasure Island (FL):

StatPearls Publishing, January 2022), https://www.ncbi.nlm.nih.gov/books/NBK459370/.

120 A. L. Brantsaeter, M. Haugen, S. O. Samuelsen, H. Torjusen, L. Trogstad, J. Alexander, P. Magnus, and H. M. Meltzer, "A Dietary Pattern Characterized by High Intake of Vegetables, Fruits, and Vegetable Oils Is Associated with Reduced Risk of Preeclampsia in Nulliparous Pregnant Norwegian Women." *J Nutr* 139, no. 6 (June 2009): 1,162–8, doi: 10.3945/jn.109.104968, epub April 15, 2009, PMID: 19369368, PMCID: PMC2682988.

121 A. M. Baker, S. Haeri, C. A. Camargo Jr., J. A. Espinola, and A. M. Stuebe, "A Nested Case-Control Study of Midgestation Vitamin D Deficiency and Risk of Severe Preeclampsia," *J Clin Endocrinol Metab* 95, no. 11 (November 2010): 5,105–9, doi: 10.1210/jc.2010-0996, epub August 18, 2010, PMID: 20719829, PMCID: PMC2968727.

122 S. Khalili, L. Amiri-Farahani, S. Haghani, A. Bordbar, A. Shojaii, and S. Pezaro, "The Effect of Pimpinella Anisum Herbal Tea on Human Milk Volume and Weight Gain in the Preterm Infant: A Randomized Controlled Clinical Trial," *BMC Complement Med Ther* 23, no. 1 (January 21, 2023 1): 19, doi: 10.1186/s12906-023-03848-6, PMID: 36681821, PMCID: PMC9862552

123 Natalie Falicz, *The Girl behind the Cape: How I Found My Depth, Voice and Value from Within* (Australia).

124 J. Tregoning, "Imperial," *Neonatal Immunology*, https://www.immunology.org/public-information/bitesized-immunology/immune-development/neonatal-immunology; T. Obukhanych, https://immunologyfordailyliving.substack.com/about.

125 www.homstudy.net.

126 https://stresslessbehealthy.com/healthy-eating-quotes/.

127 https://truemedicine.com.au/treatments/childrens-health/eczema/.

128 K. Wickens, P. Black, T. V. Stanley, E. Mitchell, C. Barthow, P. Fitzharris, G. Purdie, and J. Crane, "A Protective Effect of Lactobacillus rhamnosus HN001 against Eczema in the First 2 Years of Life Persists to Age 4 Years," *Clin Exp Allergy* 42, no. 7 (July 2012): 1,071–9, doi: 10.1111/j.1365-2222.2012.03975.x, PMID: 22702506.

129 C. Moriarty and W. Carroll, "Paracetamol: Pharmacology, Prescribing and Controversies," http://dx.doi.org/10.1136/archdischild-2014-307287 https://ep.bmj.com/content/101/6/331.long.

130 J. Rajanayagam, J. R. Bishop, P. J. Lewindon, and H. M. Evans, "Paracetamol-Associated Acute Liver Failure in Australian and New Zealand Children: High Rate of Medication Errors," http://dx.doi.org/10.1136/archdischild-2013-304902.

131 K. Mareckova, R. Marecek, L. Andryskova, M. Brazdil, and Y. S. Nikolova, "Impact of Prenatal Stress on Amygdala Anatomy in Young Adulthood: Timing and Location Matter," *Biol Psychiatry Cogn Neurosci Neuroimaging* 7, no. 2

(February 2022): 231–8, doi: 10.1016/j.bpsc.2021.07.009, epub August 3, 2021, PMID: 34358683.

132. A. Lautarescu, M. C. Craig, and V. Glover, "Prenatal Stress: Effects on Fetal and Child Brain Development," *Int Rev Neurobiol* 150 (2020): 17–40, doi: 10.1016/bs.irn.2019.11.002, epub December 14, 2019, PMID: 32204831.

133. https://truemedicine.com.au/tips/moods-mind-or-biochemistry/.

134. E. P. Davis, L. M. Glynn, F. Waffarn, and C. A. Sandman, "Prenatal Maternal Stress Programs Infant Stress Regulation," *J Child Psychol Psychiatry* 52, no. 2 (February 2011): 119–29, doi: 10.1111/j.1469-7610.2010.02314.x, epub September 20, 2010, PMID: 20854366, PMCID: PMC3010449.

135. Jeromy Johnson, "Wireless Wakeup Call," https://www.youtube.com/watch?v=F0NEaPTu9oI.

136. B. J. Houston, B. Nixon, B. V. King, G. N. De Iuliis, and R. J. Aitken, "The Effects of Radiofrequency Electromagnetic Radiation on Sperm Function," *Reproduction* 152, no. 6 (December 2016): R263–R276, doi: 10.1530/REP-16-0126, epub September 6, 2016, PMID: 27601711.

137. D. K. Li, H. Chen, J. R. Ferber et al., "Exposure to Magnetic Field Non-Ionizing Radiation and the Risk of Miscarriage: A Prospective Cohort Study," *Sci Rep* 7 (2017): 17,541, https://doi.org/10.1038/s41598-017-16623-8.

138. https://www.sciencedirect.com/topics/materials-science/oxidative-damage.

139. Ill Health from WIFI, https://sourcepointglobaloutreach.org/wp-content/uploads/2014/08/Health-Problems-from-WiFi.pdf.

140. J. E. McCredden, N. Cook, S. Weller, and V. Leach, "Wireless Technology Is an Environmental Stressor Requiring New Understanding and Approaches in Health Care," *Front Public Health* 10 (December 20, 2022): 986,315, doi: 10.3389/fpubh.2022.986315, PMID: 36605238, PMCID: PMC9809975.

141. M. N. Mead, "Nutrigenomics: The Genome-Food Interface," *Environ Health Perspect* 115, no. 12 (December 2007): A582–9, doi: 10.1289/ehp.115-a582, PMID: 18087577, PMCID: PMC2137135.

142. C. J. Carter and R. A. Blizard, "Autism Genes Are Selectively Targeted by Environmental Pollutants Including Pesticides, Heavy Metals, Bisphenol A, Phthalates and Many Others in Food, Cosmetics or Household Products," *Neurochem Int* S0197–0186, no. 16 (October 27, 2016): 30,197–8, doi: 10.1016/j.neuint.2016.10.011, epub ahead of print, PMID: 27984170.

143. Andrew Rostenberg, *Your Genius Body: A Guide for Optimizing Your Genes and Changing Your Life* (Boise).

144. https://www.healthline.com/nutrition/essential-amino-acids#how-many-are-there.

145. Henry Osiecki, *The Nutrient Bible*, 9th ed. (Australia: Orthoplex).

Keep up with the latest research in fertility, pregnancy, and antenatal care at:

https://truemedicine.com.au/

https://www.facebook.com/TrueMedicine/
https://www.linkedin.com/in/dagmar-ganser-true-medicine/

Please send me your thoughts, comments and questions as we never stop learning.

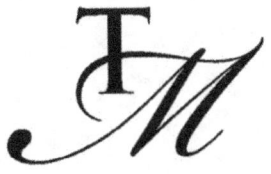

www.ingramcontent.com/pod-product-compliance
Lightning Source LLC
Chambersburg PA
CBHW050311010526
44107CB00055B/2190